PRAISE FOR
SMART PEOPLE DON'T DIET

"Since all of the data indicate that diets don't work, Dr. Markey proposes a reasonable path to good health in easy, doable steps. Dr. Markey gives insights into why we eat the foods we eat, and how we can change our inclinations so that we pick healthier choices. She suggests ways to change habits, and there are many easy-to-read tables throughout that give alternative food options. And most importantly, Dr. Markey writes about how positive feelings about our body shape and characteristics can spur us to strive for health."

—JOSEPH DIXON, PhD,
Department of Nutritional Sciences, Rutgers University

SMART PEOPLE DON'T DIET

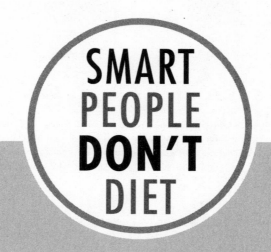

SMART
PEOPLE
DON'T
DIET

How the Latest Science
Can Help You Lose Weight
Permanently

CHARLOTTE N. MARKEY, PhD

Da Capo
LIFE
LONG

A Member of the Perseus Books Group

Designed by Brent Wilcox
Set in 11.75 point Adobe Garamond Pro by the Perseus Books Group

Library of Congress Cataloging-in-Publication Data
Markey, Charlotte N., author.
    Smart people don't diet : how psychology, common sense, and the latest science can help you lose
weight permanently / by Charlotte N. Markey, PhD. — First Da Capo Press edition.
        pages   cm
    Includes bibliographical references and index.
    ISBN 978-0-7382-1771-0 (paperback) — ISBN 978-0-7382-1772-7 (e-book)
    1. Weight loss.   2. Weight loss—Psychological aspects.   3. Self-care, Health.   I. Title.
    RM222.2.M3577 2014
    613.2'5—dc23
                                                                                      2014031432

Published by Da Capo Press
A Member of the Perseus Books Group
www.dacapopress.com

Note: The information in this book is true and complete to the best of our knowledge. This book is
intended only as an informative guide for those wishing to know more about health issues. In no way
is this book intended to replace, countermand, or conflict with the advice given to you by your own
physician. The ultimate decision concerning care should be made between you and your doctor. We
strongly recommend you follow his or her advice. Information in this book is general and is offered
with no guarantees on the part of the author or Da Capo Press. The author and publisher disclaim all
liability in connection with the use of this book. The names and identifying details of some
individuals in this book have been changed.

Da Capo Press books are available at special discounts for bulk purchases in the US by corporations,
institutions, and other organizations. For more information, please contact the Special Markets
Department at the Perseus Books Group, 2300 Chestnut Street, Suite 200, Philadelphia, PA 19103,
or call (800) 810-4145, ext. 5000, or e-mail special.markets@perseusbooks.com.
10 9 8 7 6 5 4 3 2 1

For Charlie and Grace
The best reasons I can think of to keep eating my vegetables

Note: A portion of the proceeds from sales of this book will be donated to The Food Trust (www.TheFoodTrust.org) to fund programs that facilitate education about healthy eating for children.

Download the companion app designed
to help you follow the advice in this book.
Scan the QR code or go to www.SmartenFit.com.

CONTENTS

INTRODUCTION

I Wasn't Always Smart

I've been obsessed with food for as long as I can remember. As a young girl, I was convinced I would one day be a ballerina. Of course, most little girls want to be ballerinas, but I *really* was going to be a prima ballerina. A decade in the dance world inevitably resulted in a lot of scrutiny about what I ate and what I weighed. By the age of twelve, I knew quite a bit about dieting, but that was expected as a girl auditioning to be a part of San Francisco Ballet. During the audition, I was told that I would not be admitted into the company. In fact, I was told that I would not ever make it as a dancer because I "simply did not have a dancer's body." At the time, I was crushed; today, this memory serves only to confuse me. I don't remember what I weighed back then, but I know I was nowhere near overweight. Unfortunately, my preadolescent self just assumed I was fat, and I reluctantly left ballet for more typical teenage pursuits: sports, cheerleading, boys.

Watching my weight wasn't reinforced only on the dance floor but also at home, where someone was always on a diet. I learned how to count calories before I hit puberty. And, I learned a lesson that the dance world had first introduced: watching what you ate was a normal part of life. Adolescent insecurities ramped up my interest in dieting, and it wasn't long before my obsession with food led to a dark chapter of my life. By the middle of high school, my weight was hovering below a hundred pounds and I had already achieved my adult height of five feet five inches. Fortunately, there were people who noticed when I lost weight. A high school math teacher (an intimidating man who also happened to be the school's football coach) sat me down, expressed uncharacteristic empathy, shared his own struggles with his weight, and offered sound nutritional advice. My swim coach encouraged me to be proud of my "strong legs," and a school counselor never failed to just ask me how I was doing when he saw me. My family worried, my friends provided support and encouragement, and doctors assured everyone that there was no medical explanation for my weight loss.

There was no dramatic turning point or epiphany that led me to eat more, take better care of myself, and return to a healthy weight. I became older and more mature, and I suppose I gradually came to terms with the fact that I was not being smart, I was potentially compromising my health to be thin. My story is not one of a magical moment of redemption; it's a story of a typical, insecure teenage girl who gradually learned what healthy eating entailed with some help from a nutritionist, good social support, and the pursuit of a degree in psychology.

When I began my undergraduate education at Santa Clara University, I did not plan to major in psychology. But, after taking a few classes, I was hooked. I loved that a scientific, methodical approach was available to help me understand my world better. I began to do research during my senior year of college, and—not surprising, I suppose—my initial focus was on children's eating attitudes. I applied to graduate school because I loved psychology and wanted to continue doing this research. By that time, I had moved beyond trying to merely understand myself to wanting to understand all the children, adolescents, and adults who struggle with poor body image and engage in maladaptive eating behaviors. I was lucky to receive incredible training at the Healthy Families Project (University of California, Riverside), the Children's Eating Lab (Pennsylvania State University), and the Longevity Project (University of California, Riverside) while I completed my PhD in health and developmental psychology.

In 2002, I joined the faculty at Rutgers University and developed a course called the Psychology of Eating. Many years later, I still love teaching this class, and my research at Rutgers focuses on issues ranging from romantic partners' influences on eating behaviors to parents' concerns about their children's obesity risk. For some, thinking about food, doing research about food, and teaching about food (never mind the need to eat food!) for this many years would be unappetizing, but I've never tired of the subject and don't expect that I will any time soon.

I began to think about writing this book several years ago when I was teaching my Psychology of Eating course. In the class, I spend a considerable amount of time trying to debunk myths about food, dieting, and body image for my students. Most semesters, I ask students to bring in popular diet books, and we discuss them in relation to the scientific facts about weight loss; most books don't fare well once we start digging for evidence to support their claims. It turns out, for example, that there's no scientific support for a ten-day, seventeen-day, or twenty-one-day weight loss plan, regardless of what some books claim. I've been encouraged by my students, who tell me that what they learn in my class is life changing and that they wish that they had known this information years ago. Time and time again, students report giving up on fad diets in favor of the gradual, sustainable, healthy approach to weight loss and weight management I offer in this book. In addition to my students, I continue to be inspired by the latest science and research, which contradicts the avalanche of inaccurate information out there and offers sound information about eating, weight, and body image.

Outside the classroom, when I tell people that I am a health psychologist who studies eating behaviors and body image, they often have a lot of questions for me. Surprisingly often (at least I'm always surprised), they start to tell me about a new diet they are trying. Favorites among people I've encountered lately seem to be the Paleo diets, Mediterranean diets, and low-carb approaches (that trend just doesn't want to die, apparently!). I'm always a bit stumped as to what to say to people when they want to talk about these diets. There are thousands of diet books and diet plans available at any given time, and many of these plans offer some reasonable advice about weight loss. Unfortunately, as my students and I have spent considerable time exploring, the vast majority of them also offer some really terrible advice.

This is not a subjective statement. Other diet plans often offer advice that is not supported by science. In fact, their advice often contradicts scientific evidence. Sometimes, their claims are so egregious, I wonder how they are even legal. As it turns out, there isn't a "book police" or a "diet plan investigative team" out there somewhere in the world evaluating the claims made by other folks who offer advice about weight loss. In fact, in the process of working on this book, I was even warned that no one really cares about science; people just want to lose weight *fast*.

If only fast worked.

Unfortunately, fast weight loss often results in fast weight gain. It's unfair but true. Many scientists, doctors, nutritionists, and psychologists understand that dieting often makes dieters gain weight rather than lose it, because nothing done for only a few days or weeks can have a long-term effect. Not only that—being on a diet is a miserable experience for most people.

So, What Does Work?

The approach to weight management that I prescribe in this book is not a typical diet. I won't be telling you exactly what, when, or how much to eat. It's not that restrictive, and it's not a quick fix. But here's the thing—it works. All of the information is supported by psychology, common sense, or science—and in most cases all three. You probably already know a lot about the advice that I will offer. For example, you know that eating less will help you to lose weight. But, do you know how to do this in a way that is sustainable? As a health psychologist, I can tell you there is *nothing* you can do for *only* a few days or weeks that will have any effect on your long-term weight loss or health.

So if this isn't a diet book, what is it? This book presents a different approach: a way to think about and change your eating and activity habits for the rest of your life. Based on what I've learned personally, studied scientifically, and teach my students, I've created a plan that addresses the psychology of weight gain and offers proven, smart strategies for healthful, *sustainable* weight loss and management, with specific advice about eating well, losing weight, and keeping it off for the rest of your life.

This book provides a 3-phase plan that offers you:

- **A psychological approach** to weight loss and maintenance that will not make you miserable.
- **A commonsense approach** to sustaining weight loss for the long term, including the tools you need to be an educated consumer and make good decisions regarding your eating and activity habits.
- **The information you need** to evaluate your own habits and a week-by-week plan to make gradual, sustainable lifestyle changes.
- **Positive advice** for getting "back on the wagon" without guilt, should you ever find yourself succumbing to unhealthy habits in the future.
- **A scientifically proven** way to feel your best at a healthy and attractive weight.

My ultimate goal is to change the way you think about food forever. The title says it all—smart people don't diet. What you hold in your hands is a diet book only in that when you finish it, I hope you don't ever think of going on a diet ever again.

Note: This book was written with all people in mind—those who want to lose five pounds, those who want to lose fifty-five pounds, and those who just want to eat better and improve their health. However, before beginning any dietary or physical activity regimen, it is recommended that you confer with your primary care physician. Further, if you are morbidly obese, need to lose a great deal of weight, and time is not on your side, this book can help you, but it is especially important for you to be under the supervision of a physician, and you should consider consulting a nutritionist as well.

Just *Don't*
Do It

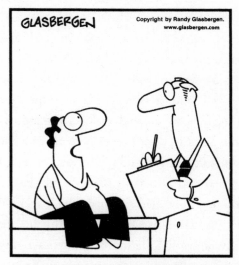

"Eat less and exercise more? That's the
most ridiculous fad diet I've heard of yet!"

When it comes to weight loss, there's no lack of fad
diets promising fast results. But such diets limit your
nutritional intake, can be unhealthy, and tend to fail
in the long run.

Centers for Disease Control and Prevention

A s I finished teaching my Psychology of Eating class this semester, one of my students wrote,

> As an on-the-go college student who wishes she had the time to lose a few pounds and be fit, a promise like "Lose 20 lbs in 2 weeks!" sounds so enticing. Just this past winter I considered doing a detox diet. This class was my first exposure to the psychological aspects of dieting, and I can honestly say that I will never consider a short-term type diet again, especially if it makes bogus promises to change my life. There's no way of getting around the fact that we need healthy lifestyles in order to have healthy bodies and minds.

It is feedback like this that led me to write *Smart People Don't Diet*.

We aren't necessarily born smart when it comes to dieting, but *we can become smart*. And I'm certainly not suggesting that because you have gone on a diet that you lack brainpower. If that were the case, then I just succeed in insulting the majority of adults (including me), who have dieted to lose weight at some point in their lives. If you are one of these individuals, let me guess the outcome of your diet. You lost a few pounds at the start, but then within a year you gained all of the weight back. Within a year of the failed diet, you probably tried another, which also failed. I don't know this about you because I'm a psychic; I know this because I've been there and I'm a scientist who studies dieting. Dieting is actually one of the worst things you can do if you are trying to lose weight. You will soon learn that *smart people don't diet* when they want to achieve long-term weight loss.

Men and women all over the world go on diets all the time. In fact, about 90 percent of women and upward of 70 percent of men in the US report dieting. Why do so many people diet? Obviously, they want to lose weight, and dieting seems like the solution. However, it is questionable how well these diets actually work. Given the rising rates of global obesity, it seems pretty clear that these diets are not causing people to get any thinner. Did you ever think that maybe there is another way?

In this chapter you will learn . . .
- To think about weight loss as a long-term goal
- How not to fall for the diet fads and, instead, focus on scientific evidence when making choices about weight loss and weight management
- Why you can both "eat to live" and "live to eat"

This book presents a different approach: a way for you to think about and change your eating and physical activity habits for the rest of your life. However, this book is as much about what you *should* do as it is about what you *shouldn't*. This is important because what most people do to lose weight doesn't work—at least not in the long term. My goal is for you to think about weight management as a long-term endeavor. I'll admit that probably sounds daunting. However, I will lay out 3 phases for revamping your eating and activity habits. My goal is to change the way you think about food and weight management forever. I want to empower you to make smart choices that enable you to enjoy food and maintain a healthy weight.

Before reading any further, it is important that you think about *why* you picked up this book in the first place. I'm guessing that you aren't happy with your current weight. Most likely, you want to lose weight, get in shape, or improve your health. Maybe you want to achieve all three of these goals. It's possible that you have a pair of jeans that you wish you could still fit into (and still be able to breathe) or you have an upcoming wedding or school reunion for which you'd like to look your best. Perhaps, as you start to feel the effects of aging, you realize the necessity of taking care of your body more than you used to—especially if you want to be around to see your children and grandchildren reach particular milestones. Although some of these goals may be more meaningful to you than others, there is really no bad reason to want to maintain an optimal weight and improve your overall health. But it is important to keep these goals in mind. Remind yourself regularly *why* you care about losing weight or maintaining a healthy weight. Reread sections of this book that especially motivate you. Talk with your family and friends about this new approach to weight loss and weight management. Make it a part of your life, not something that you do temporarily in preparation for swimsuit season.

The approach to weight loss and weight management that I prescribe in this book is not a diet. In fact, my entire approach implores you to just *don't* do it—don't diet! In this book, there are no gimmicks and no fads. I offer information that is supported by science. I've also incorporated common sense, anecdotes, interviews with experts, and other forms of wisdom to support the claims I make. My goal is to teach you how to be smart about these issues by understanding what researchers such as me know about healthy weight management (tip: fasting to fit into a pair of jeans is not supported by any research!).

Why Evidence-Based Advice Is Important

Everybody eats, so everybody thinks they are experts on eating. We may all have "gut instincts" as to the best way to lose weight, but it is important to consider what science has to say about the topic. The healthiest approach to eating is not a matter of opinion. Psychologists like me have been doing research about eating and weight loss for over a hundred years, and thousands of studies about these issues have been published. Scientists in related fields such as nutrition, medicine, and community health have also been studying and publishing about these issues for a very long time. And yet it seems that the most marketable and even outlandish ideas are what get the most attention when it comes to weight loss—not necessarily the ideas that are really going to work! Just because you would like to lose twenty pounds in two weeks does not mean that this is realistic. However, people sell outrageous ideas like this in various diet books and plans because that is what people want to buy.

In this book, I will summarize what is known from decades of research in an accessible and easy-to-read format. I'll talk about the evidence that supports what I advise so that you can become a smart consumer of all of the information you may encounter about dieting and weight loss from today forward. Advertisements and the media make a lot of enticing claims; I want you to be critical of this media information so that you no longer find yourself struggling to eat well. My goal is to empower you to maintain a healthy weight for the rest of your life. I will explain why diets don't work, why it is often difficult to lose weight, and what you can do that *will* work. This isn't my opinion; this is a fact echoed by researchers, doctors, and even the Centers for Disease Control and Prevention (CDC), which warns that weight loss isn't about dieting but about "an ongoing lifestyle that includes long-term changes in daily eating and exercise habits."[1]

What Is Weight Management?

You may be starting to notice that I tend to refer to my approach as "weight loss and weight management." How is this different from dieting? I use the term "weight management" because my approach provides you with a means to not only lose weight but *maintain* a weight you are happy with for the rest of your life. Literally, I mean how you will manage your weight. I realize that the word "manage" may sound a bit like I'm proposing that you approach eating and physical activity behaviors as a "job" you must do, that we all must do. Just like we have various jobs and activities we perform each day, we should take care of ourselves by eating well and being active every day (okay, most days). This will make us healthier, happier, and better able to contribute to our communities (as opposed to "costing" society resources; more on this point in Chapter 10). Despite the connotations of the term "job," you will not find that a smart approach to weight management ultimately results in changes to your life that feel like a lot of work.

Managing your weight is a job in some ways analogous to maintaining good hygiene and grooming practices. I think it is safe to assume that most people spend at least an hour a day bathing, brushing their teeth, doing their hair, picking out clothes, and getting dressed. Although these tasks take time, you would not forgo them (at least not for too many days, I hope). Weight management is comparable in that it may take some time each day, but it is about taking care of yourself. Many people—especially women—are quick to think that spending time on themselves is a "luxury" that they can't afford. They often have other people to look out for, and they put themselves last on their long "to do" lists. However, weight management is not just about losing weight and being skinny or attractive; it is about health. It is not a luxury; it is a necessity. Once you get in the habit of shopping for nutritious foods, planning healthy meals, and exercising, you will not forgo these tasks. Further, you should not feel guilty when you take this time for yourself. When you allow the time and energy required to manage your own weight, not only do you benefit but your loved ones will as well. Shopping for fresh produce now means everyone in your household may get more of the nutrients they need from healthy fruit and veggies later. A little more time at the gym now may mean more time to play with your grandchildren later. Weight management is a win-win for you and your loved ones.

When you hear the word "diet," you probably think of a short-term (e.g., a week, a month, etc.), strict program of eating intended to reduce your weight. Smart people don't diet because they know that sustainable weight loss and management is not a temporary pursuit. When I use the term "diet" in this book, I'm usually referring to the food and drink that you regularly consume or the dietary habits that you maintain across time. My advice is not merely about a regimen that will help you lose weight this week or this month but how you should *always* eat for the rest of your life. A key component to managing your weight is to not focus on the short term but to always think long-term when making changes to your eating and activity habits.

The second day of a diet is always easier than the first. By the second day, you're off of it.

—**Jackie Gleason**

Why Thinking Long-Term Matters So Much

Maintaining a desired weight for the rest of your life may seem like a lofty goal, but it is possible. Of course, changes in our bodies that accompany aging, including our hormone and activity levels, may make it difficult to maintain the same exact optimal weight for the rest of our lives. However, this approach to weight management allows us to make adjustments as the circumstances of our lives change. And, as you'll see, this really isn't that difficult to do.

One of the essential ingredients in my recipe for weight management (if you'll humor the cooking reference) is to make changes to your eating and activity patterns that you believe you can maintain *for the rest of your life*. When people lose weight they want to keep it off. Gaining it back is typically viewed as a sort of personal failure. However, what you may not realize is that this failure is almost inevitable.[2] If you followed a plan that required you to eliminate something from your diet—say sugar or carbs—that you didn't really intend to continue to eliminate from your diet for the rest of your life, then it was predictable that when you added these foods back to your diet you would gain weight. Let's say it is April, and you are concerned about the coming bathing suit season, so you cut out all sweets and desserts from your diet and lose ten pounds. You might be very happy about this weight loss—and it's all from eliminating "bad foods" from your diet that don't offer a lot of nutritional value. However, after a while, you probably will want to eat desserts—at least every once in a while. So, as you add these foods back to your diet, you will gradually add the pounds back to your body and your summer body will soon return to your winter body. The complete elimination of a desired food item from your diet is never going to be an effective long-term approach to weight management.[3]

Of course, not all diet plans suggest that you cut particular foods out of your diet entirely. Instead, some programs will require you to make temporary changes to your eating and exercise habits. This is the same problem as before: unless you are willing to make these changes forever, temporarily altering your activity level or diet will not result in sustainable weight loss. The goal of this book is to offer advice that you can integrate into your existing lifestyle for years. That is, you tailor the "diet" to fit into your life rather than changing who you are to fit the diet. I want *you* to select the foods that you like and can envision continuing to eat for the rest of your life. If you follow my advice, it is unlikely that you will be eating chips and cake for all of your meals. But you will be "allowed" to eat chips and cake. This advice also holds true for making physical activity a regular part of your life. It doesn't particularly matter if you walk, run, lift weights, or learn to ride a unicycle. What matters is that you incorporate exercise that you like and believe that you will be able to continue to do. I said it above, but I'll continue to say it throughout this book: make changes to your eating and exercise habits that you can make for the rest of your life!

MICHAEL'S *Story*

As a guy, I had never been overly concerned about my weight or what I was eating. I simply didn't think about food. Then one day I found out that my weight and height clearly placed me in the overweight category. Overweight? Me? Although I still saw myself as a twentysomething athletic guy, I had to get real. I was a father of two in my late thirties who was no longer in shape. After hearing about Dr. Markey's Smart Diet and reading the scientific literature it was based on, I decided to give it a try. After recording what I ate (and trying not to cheat), I was shocked at how many items I was eating that really were not that healthy for me. After seeing this pattern I selected one item to reduce—I substituted diet soda or water for my usual regular soda. After a couple of weeks, I didn't miss the soda. I then selected another item to reduce and then another and another. This was an unhurried process, and with each item eliminated or cut back I would ask myself, "Can I do this forever?" I didn't want to just lose weight and then gain it back a year later!

As my new eating style progressed, I didn't notice my weight changing that much. It was a slow process—but it wasn't painful. After a few months, a coworker asked me whether I was losing weight and whether I was on a diet. I was happy to tell her that I was losing weight but that I wasn't on a diet—I was just eating healthier. For the past two years, I have been eating healthy and even exercising (something that just kind of happened once I started to eat better). I have lost more than thirty-five pounds, and, given that I am totally content with what I am eating, I can't imagine that I will gain it back.

~Michael, AGE THIRTY-NINE, PROFESSOR

What Are Your Other Options?

It sometimes seems like each person you meet is either on a new diet or is adopting the newest quick-fix approach to weight loss. Perhaps one of your friend's experiences of success on a Mediterranean diet plan has motivated you to try it. Maybe you've been thinking of trying a low-carb diet or a Paleo diet. Do you know what these diets entail or whether they are even effective in the long run? I'll save you some of the hassle of figuring out whether my advice will be helpful and effective for you by making some comparisons between my approach and some other diets. Although there are a countless number of diet plans, the following table features the central elements of some of the more popular ones contrasted with the approach offered in this book.

	APPROACH	DIETARY RECOMMENDATIONS	EVIDENCE AND EVALUATION
Paleo	This approach is based upon eating wholesome, contemporary foods from the food groups available to our hunter-gatherer ancestors during the Paleolithic era.	Emphasis on fresh meats (e.g., preferably grass-produced or free-ranging beef, pork, lamb, poultry, and game meat, fish and other seafood), fruits, vegetables, seeds, nuts, and healthful oils (e.g., olive oil). Dairy products, cereal, grains, legumes, refined sugars and processed foods are not allowed.	Elimination of dairy products is a poor choice for many people because they are an important source of calcium and protein, although this may facilitate weight loss.[1] Avoidance of refined sugars and processed foods is nutritionally advantageous but may be difficult to maintain in the current food environment.[2] According to the Mayo Clinic, research examining long-term weight loss and health is not available.[3]
Low-Carb	Different approaches include the Atkins Diet, the South Beach Diet and the Dukan Diet. They typically prescribe elimination of all carbohydrates (esp. bread and fruit products) initially with the gradual inclusion of some of these foods. A low-carb diet is thought to lower insulin levels in the body, which may reduce fat storage and weight.	Emphasis is on protein consumption (i.e., meat and cheese) as 30–50 percent of diet. Reduce (or eliminate, depending on the specific low-carb diet) fruits, milk, nuts, grains, seeds, legumes, and starchy vegetables.	Reduction of nonnutritive carbohydrates (e.g., white bread) is supported by nutritionists.[4] Individuals who engage in low-carbohydrate dieting typically lose about the same amount of weight as other dieters. Dieters indicate that maintaining a low-carb approach is difficult long-term.[5] Some research suggests that low-carb dieters can expect a nine-pound weight loss after two years.[6]
Mediterranean	Often referred to as a "heart healthy" diet based on European (e.g., Italian, Greek, Spanish) approaches to eating.	Emphasis on plant foods such as vegetables, fruits, beans, whole grains, nuts, olives, and olive oil. Moderate amounts of (low-fat) cheese, yogurt, poultry, and eggs. Most of the foods on the plan are fresh and seasonal whole foods (not processed). Only small amounts of saturated fat, sodium, sweets, and red meat are part of the plan. A focus on "good fats" (primarily from olive oil) and moderate red wine consumption.	Evidence shows that the Mediterranean diet reduces risk of cardiovascular disease and may increase longevity.[7] If caloric intake is less than the individual's intake prior to adopting this diet and physical activity is incorporated, weight loss is likely. Concerns for sustainability include the cost of foods (like fish), time for preparation of foods, and regular avoidance of sweets.

| Long-Term Weight Management (i.e., a smart approach) | Focus on understanding the psychology of eating for health and eating for life. Initial goal is to record eating and physical activity behaviors. Gradual dietary and physical activity changes introduced one week at a time. Emphasis on education about healthful food choices. Eating and physical activity are customized by the individual. | Enjoy all desired foods in moderation. Learn to make dietary changes so that healthy options are incorporated into regular diet. No foods are completely "off limits." | Inclusion of desired foods and moderate, gradual approach to weight loss is supported by countless scientific studies.[8] Avoiding complete restriction of specific foods is supported by decades of research.[9] Focus on a long-term approach is supported by psychological research and the CDC. (Evidence for this approach is presented throughout this book.) |

[1]Zemel, M. B., Thompson, W., Milstead, A., Morris, K., & Campbell, P. (2012). Calcium and dairy acceleration of weight and fat loss during energy restriction in obese adults. *Obesity: A Research Journal, 12,* 582–589. doi: 10.1038/oby.2004.67

[2]Brownell, K., & Battle Horgen, K. (2004). *Food fight: The inside story of the food industry, America's obesity crisis, and what we can do about it.* McGraw-Hill, New York.

[3]Frassetto, L. A., Schloetter, M., Mietus-Sydner, M., Morris, R. C., Sebastian, A. (2009). Metabolic and physiologic improvements from consuming a Paleolithic, hunter-gatherer type diet. *European Journal of Clinical Nutrition, 63,* 947–955.

[4]Harvard School of Public Health. (n.d.). *The nutrition source: Carbohydrates.* Retrieved February 10, 2013, http://www.hsph.harvard.edu/nutritionsource/carbohydrates/

[5]Ebbeling, C. B., Leidig, M. M., Feldman, H. A., Lovesky, M. M., & Ludwig, D. S. (2007). Effects of a low-glycemic load vs. low-fat diet in obese young adults: A randomized trial. *Journal of the American Medical Association, 297,* 2092–2102.

[6]Mayo Clinic. (2011, October 11). Healthy lifestyle: Weight loss. Retrieved February 1, 2013, http://www.mayoclinic.com/health/low-carb-diet/NU00279/NSECTIONGROUP=2

[7]Knoops, K. T. B., de Groot, L. C. P., Kromhout, D., Perrin, A., Moreiras-Varela, O., Menotti, A., & van Staveren, W. A. (2004). Mediterranean diet, lifestyle factors, and 10-year mortality in elderly European men and women. *Journal of the American Medical Association, 12,* 1433–1439.

[8]CDC. (2011, August 17). Healthy weight—it's not a diet, it's a lifestyle! Retrieved February 11, 2013, http://www.cdc.gov/healthyweight/losing_weight/index.html; US Department of Health and Human Services. (2005, August). *Aim for a healthy weight.* Retrieved February 10, 2013, http://www.nhlbi.nih.gov/health/public/heart/obesity/aim_hwt.pdf

[9]CDC (2011).

At the Extreme

In addition to the popular diet plans that I discuss above, there are more extreme approaches to weight loss that have received attention in recent years. I describe these alternatives to the approach offered in this book *not* to recommend them. In fact, I hope that as you read more of this book you come to understand how ineffective most of these approaches are likely to be. To understand what you *should* do to maintain a healthy weight, it is important that you understand what you *shouldn't* do. Often, what you shouldn't do is quite popular, so let's review some of the more extreme options.

As obesity rates have risen in the United States and around the world, surgical approaches to treating obesity have become increasingly popular. There are many surgeries utilized to promote weight loss including gastric bypass, vertical banded gastroplasty, and adjustable gastric banding (LapBand). These procedures all involve restricting the amount of space in the stomach, making it impossible for individuals to eat as much as they did previously. The success rates of these procedures (about 60 percent of obese and morbidly obese individuals have been found to experience excellent results five years postsurgery) make them a reasonable option to consider for severely obese individuals.[4] Many celebrities and other folks who garner considerable media attention, from Al Roker to Star Jones to most recently Chris Christie, have had success using surgical weight loss procedures. Their striking before and after photos no doubt encourage many to consider surgical approaches to weight loss. However, I'm hesitant to recommend surgery for two reasons. First, individuals can, theoretically, restrict what they eat without undergoing surgery. Second, these procedures are not risk-free. The National Association for Weight Loss Surgery reports that about 20 percent of individuals who undergo weight-loss surgery experience complications.[5]

If surgery isn't a risk-free quick fix for weight loss, perhaps there's a pill or potion you can take. One advertised option is a product called Sensa, which is marketed as something that you sprinkle on your food (almost like salt); do nothing else and lose weight. Sensa's web page suggests that the product is backed by scientific evidence, and it even provides a link to an abstract describing a clinical trial. The problem with this research is that a lot of important details are missing. There is no mention of following up with participants to determine whether weight loss using the product is maintained. There appears to be no accounting for participants' other diet or exercise behaviors that may also affect weight loss. And the research itself was not published in a peer-reviewed journal but was presented as a poster at a conference in Prague.[6] (For those who don't know, the standards for presenting a poster at a conference are pretty low, as this is where many researchers present the early stages of their research before formally publishing the results in a peer-reviewed journal.) Additionally, there are ethical issues with this research, because the primary author of this study examining the effectiveness of Sensa is also the person who is selling Sensa to the public. Thus, although their website suggests that "non-caloric tastant crystals sprinkled on food prior to consumption" leads to less hunger, less food eaten, and weight loss, I remain very skeptical. The Federal Trade Commission shares my skepticism and recently settled a $26.5 million lawsuit with Sensa for making unfounded weight-loss claims and misleading endorsements. Of course, most misleading diet claims are never challenged; you have to be a smart consumer to avoid falling prey to them.

Another "medical" approach to weight loss that received some media attention in the past year is the feeding tube diet. This diet is what it sounds like. Individuals have a feeding tube inserted into their nose that goes down their throat. They remain attached to a pump that feeds them throughout the day. They don't eat any real food, and they do seem to lose weight. Dr. Oliver DiPietro created this "K-E," or feeding tube, diet and claims that his diet is not extreme.[7] But, unless you are willing to have a feeding tube inserted in your nose for the rest of your life, it seems likely that you will eventually gain back all the weight lost while using the feeding tube. This sort of an approach capitalizes on many people's misconception about weight loss, that when you lose weight it literally "goes away." But losing weight is not like losing a camera on the subway, which you have little hope of ever finding again. Weight lost can easily return. Unless you keep doing whatever you were doing to lose weight in the first place, you will gain weight back. Regular "treatments" with a feeding tube may allow for persistent weight loss, but it seems like an odd trade-off to be attractively thin yet have a feeding tube in your nose on a regular basis.

Perhaps a bit less extreme than the feeding tube diet are increasingly popular juicing, cleansing, detoxing, and fasting diets. Usually, these approaches—touted as not only weight loss prescriptions but as means of purifying the body and improving health—include a few days of water and juice consumption with no solid food allowed. Unless I'm scheduled for a colonoscopy the next day and I have strict doctor's orders to avoid solid foods, there is no way that I'm going to even attempt something that requires forgoing real food. Further, what folks seem to forget is that our kidneys and liver have a job to do—they remove the toxins from our bodies. So, we do not need to "detox" or "cleanse" because our bodies do this naturally every day.

My own personal interest in solids aside, there has been something alluring about these approaches since the 1990s when the Master Cleanse (the 1940s grandfather of cleansing) was repackaged and mass marketed. Many people, including celebrities, claim that a juicing, cleansing regimen makes them feel more focused and "more alive." You don't need to be a rocket scientist to figure out that you will lose weight if you consume an extremely low-calorie diet (in many cases, cleansing regimens require less than 1,000 calories a day for a limited period of time). However, the downsides associated with these approaches to weight loss far outweigh any potential benefits. First of all, weight loss from a reduced-calorie diet will not be sustained once caloric intake is increased. Call it juicing, cleansing, or detoxifying if you will, but if you go from eating 2,500 calories a day to consuming (not eating) 1,000 calories a day, you will lose weight. Then you'll get hungry after a few days, you'll go back to eating 2,500 calories a day, and you'll gain any weight you lost. Second, how does your body respond to these fluctuations in weight? Basically, your body fears starving and slows your metabolism down, which is not conducive to long-term weight loss (I'll discuss metabolism more in the next chapter). Third, the fancier your regimen, the more it is likely to cost you. The BluePrintCleanse approach costs upward of fifty-five dollars a day.[8] You can buy a lot of real, good, healthy food for that kind of money! And, finally, these concoctions can be far from delicious. Writing for the *New York Times,* Judith Newman described the green juice she included in a three-day regimen: "like drinking everything bad that ever happened to [her] in high school."[9]

Perhaps some of these approaches sound crazy to you. You may be thinking, "I would never do that!" However, are they really all that different from cutting out all carbs from your diet? Or committing to forgo chocolate? Is drinking some thick, green juice for three "meals" a day for a week better or worse for you than a regular calorie-restriction diet? As a health psychologist who is well aware of the steady rise in obesity rates and of the poor prognosis of dieting, I have spent years studying how weight loss can be achieved. The major deficit I find in other approaches to weight loss is that none of them provide a reasonable plan that individuals can stick with for many years. Even weight-loss surgery is far from 100 percent effective. To lose weight and keep it off, individuals must find an approach that they can stick with for the rest of their lives. In other words, diets don't work. A scientific, evidence-based approach to long-term weight management does.

One cannot think well, love well, sleep well, if one has not dined well.

—Virginia Woolf

Stop the Guilt; Food Is Fun

Although I recommend changing your eating habits to enhance your health and encourage weight loss (as needed), I never want you to lose sight of the fact that food is fun. For too many people food is a source of angst and guilt; it is something they wish they could do without. This is truly sad because it leaves people unable to enjoy one of life's greatest pleasures—food! One of the greatest joys of my childhood was baking with my mother. My mom and I made cookies, homemade jam from the apricots in our backyard, and whatever sort of cake I wanted for my birthday each year. My mom's carrot cake with cream cheese frosting was blissful. It is sad that as we get older many of us not only start to avoid such foods but actually start to fear them. This fear began for me when I was barely a teenager, and carrot cake would have been a guilt-inducing indulgence. I would have silently sworn to eat next to nothing the following day. Fortunately, in my early adulthood, I relearned to find pleasure in food. I eat it, I enjoy it, and I share food with my family and friends without regret. It has truly changed my life for the better, and I don't weigh any more because of it.

My goal in writing this book is not to make eating a chore or to suggest a plan that leaves you feeling deprived. In fact, research suggests that if you completely deprive yourself of foods that you really enjoy, you are likely to overeat those foods when you do allow yourself to eat them.[10] I don't want you to think of some foods as "good" and some foods as "bad." I don't always eat healthily. In fact, I probably eat plenty of foods that fall on some people's "bad" list. However, I do enjoy food, and I feel strongly that food should be a source of pleasure and not guilt. Food is not just about the nutrients we consume but the parties where food is served, the cakes that mark celebrations, and even the cocktails we cry into after a bad day.

The trick of course is to enjoy food without overindulging regularly. This requires many people to change their approach to eating. Some people have talked about "mindful eating" or "savoring," which usually entails eating slowly and focusing on the pleasure derived from eating; both of these concepts share some similarities to the approach that I take in this book.[11] However, I don't believe that you need to have a philosophical approach to eating to enjoy food. Just look at how little kids eat. They typically make a mess and get food all over themselves and their surroundings, but they also typically exhibit true enjoyment of eating. It may not be culturally acceptable for us to eat with our hands and leave a meal with food in our hair and on our clothes, but that doesn't mean that we can't appreciate food as something that can really, truly be fun.

How to Use This Book

Some of the chapters in this book offer specific advice about how you can eat well, lose weight, and maintain a healthy weight (Chapters 3, 5, and 7). Other chapters provide the evidence or the basis for the advice that I'm offering (Chapters 2, 4, 8, 9, and 10). An additional few chapters discuss important related issues including body image (Chapter 4), physical activity (Chapter 6), and the "big picture" concerning healthy weight management (Chapter 10). These chapters are organized in such a way that it will make the most sense to read them sequentially, but if you want to skip around, you will still understand my approach to weight loss and management with little trouble. Most importantly, I want you to realize that this book represents the amalgamation of many psychologists' and other scientists' research, my experiences as a professor of the psychology of eating, my experiences as a researcher of eating behaviors and body image, and my own personal experiences of weight management. Consider today to be the beginning of your journey to long-term healthy weight management.

- Think long-term if you want to lose weight and not gain it back.
- Fads are dangerous; you want to focus on a healthy approach.
- A healthy, gradual approach to weight management is not only scientifically supported but likely to be easier and more effective in the long term.
- A back-to-basics, evidence-based approach will lead you to permanent weight loss.

STAY
SMART

Why Diets Don't Work

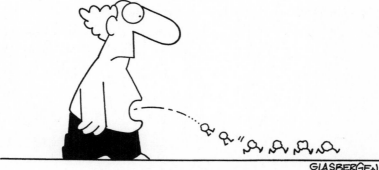

**After two weeks of dieting,
Larry's fat cells decided to go out for a pizza.**

The dieting industry is the only profitable business
in the world with a 98 percent failure rate.

Federal Trade Commission

C hances are you know one or maybe two people who have been successful at losing weight—and keeping it off. You probably know many more who haven't been successful. Perhaps you are one such person who continues to be locked in an endless struggle with your up-and-down weight. If so, this is nothing to feel embarrassed about or ashamed of—it happens to the best of us, because the diet trap is so easy to fall into. Every week it seems that a new diet book or approach to weight loss becomes readily available. Most of us find these strategies attractive—delicious even. They often suggest that weight loss is not only possible but easy—as long as we follow the prescribed plan. Although these plans are initially enticing, more often than not we soon realize that they don't live up to their promises.

My plan doesn't have a seven-day guarantee, nor is it a short-term endeavor that promises easy, rapid weight loss. But here's what my plan can promise you that others cannot: it really works.

If you approach a diet as a short-term solution to weight loss, you are likely to end up heavier (and less happy) than when you started. This is why most diets don't work. One of the most striking findings from decades of research about diets is that diets cause weight *gain* as often as they contribute to weight loss. One of the best predictors of obesity is—can you guess?—a history of dieting!

Dieting Is Not Fun

I've yet to hear someone on a diet proclaim, "I'm having a great time!" And yet, we continue to do it. According to my research, the vast majority of people diet at some point. Why do we do it? We're motivated by the outcome (pounds lost!) that we desperately hope and often expect to experience. We imagine ourselves thinner, more attractive, healthier, and happier. These are powerful motivators and the dieting industry knows it. Jenny Craig promises to make you "feel like new. Feel like you."[1] Nutrisystem's web page asks, "Ready to take the first step towards

In this chapter you will learn . . .

- The reasons why most diets are ineffective
- Why dieting is often a miserable and counterproductive experience
- Why my approach to weight management is an effective method for losing weight, keeping it off, and enjoying food

a healthier, happier you today?"[2] Dr. Michael Moreno's 17-Day Diet Plan suggests that you will never feel tired, hungry, or deprived while burning "twice as many calories as the average person."[3] Who doesn't want to feel this way? Unfortunately, dieting hardly ever inspires happy feelings; instead, it is likely to make even the most upbeat person pretty miserable.

The first thing you lose on a diet is your sense of humor.

—**Author Unknown**

Dieting Makes You Cranky

What happens when you go on a diet? Typically, you make a firm decision to eat less bad food and more healthy food. Starting tomorrow! You commit to carrot sticks over chips. Apples over donuts. In fact, you will give up sugar from now on—forever. Add to that carbs. And fat. Sound familiar?

The problem is that, if you're like me, you like chips, donuts, carbs, and fat! You don't really want to give up these foods. And, now that you've given everything up, you're cranky. And you're actually hungry. Your internal feelings of hunger are biologically driven signals that remind you to eat. When you get this signal and what you truly want to eat is a hamburger, a healthy salad is not going to feel like a satisfactory substitute. So you feel deprived and even crankier.

One of the first studies that set out to understand the link between food deprivation and mood examined conscientious objectors during World War II.[4] These people consented to participate in a semistarvation "diet" for six months with the aim of reducing their current body weight by 25 percent. All of the participants started out in excellent physical and mental health and were monitored to ensure that they stayed healthy and safe. They were all able, with a great deal of support and instruction, to stick to the prescribed low-calorie diet. But that was expected. The most striking part of this study was what happened to the participants' psychological state as a result of being in the study. They became obsessed with food. They began to think about food much more than they had before taking part in the study. Some of the participants even began to dream about food. The participants commented on an inability to focus on regular activities. They also became more socially withdrawn, depressed, and irritable. They lost interest in sex, and at least one was said to have participated in self-mutilation. In other words, they became extremely cranky.

Most dieters don't set out to lose 25 percent of their body weight in six months, but many will experience side effects similar to those experienced by the participants in the semistarvation study. Individuals who participate in very low-calorie diets (i.e., less than 1,000 kcal per day) are especially likely to experience noticeable mood swings and may experience anxiety, irritability, anger, frustration, depression, and even suicidal thoughts.[5] Dieters whose moods are monitored in studies report being in relatively good moods on the days they are allowed to "cheat" on their diets and being irritable and in bad moods on the days that they stick to a prescribed low-calorie diet. This probably makes a lot of sense to you—right? We are cranky when we're not "allowed" to eat what we want, and when we are free to eat as we please we feel good (at least initially, until the guilt sets in). So, the trick is to lose your unwanted pounds without feeling deprived or cranky.

There is a charm about the forbidden that makes it unspeakably desirable.

—Mark Twain

The More You Think About Dieting, the More You Want to Eat

Modern studies confirm the findings from the semistarvation study and elaborate on them. When you believe you are supposed to limit the amount or types of foods you eat, you usually want to eat only those foods—and a lot of them. So if you tell yourself that you will not eat pasta or bread, you will soon find yourself desiring spaghetti pomodoro with a baguette. Food preoccupation is an almost inevitable result of dieting.[6] Psychologists call this phenomenon—the preoccupation with a thought that results from attempts to suppress or avoid that thought—"ironic processing." This idea first became famous when a social psychologist, Daniel Wegner, did a series of studies that have since become known as the "white bear studies."[7] In these studies, Wegner asked his participants to avoid all thoughts of a white bear. They were asked to put any image or ideas about white bears out of their minds. White bears at a zoo, polar bears. Big or small, tame or wild, they were told, whatever you do, do not think about white bears. And, what do you think happened? The participants couldn't stop thinking about white bears! I bet you weren't thinking about white bears when you started reading this chapter. But, I bet you're thinking of a white bear now! Now try to put the image of chocolate cake out of your mind. You are not "allowed" to have chocolate cake, so put the image of it out of your mind. In fact, don't think about anything involving chocolate. Can you do it? My guess is that your thoughts are now all about chocolate. You might be thinking of a big cake with lots of frosting or maybe a smaller cupcake. Images of candy bars and Tootsie Rolls are now dancing in your head as your mouth starts to water. The point is, the more you try not to think about chocolate cake, the more you focus your mental energy on it. Ironic, isn't it?

It could be argued that many of us are preoccupied with food even when we are not trying to lose weight because in this country we're constantly surrounded by palatable, easy-to-shove-into-our-mouths food options. Whether it's on-the-go foods like pizza or hamburgers or a fancy coffee drink with piles of whipped cream, in our industrialized world, food is all around us. So many of us spend more time than we care to admit (me included) thinking about what we will eat next. And when we try not to think about food and are committed to avoiding certain foods, we set ourselves up for failure.

Attempts to avoid food are different from attempts to avoid tobacco products, alcohol, or drugs. Many addicts successfully give up smoking, drinking, or drugs by avoiding these substances all together. They are even more likely to successfully recover from their addiction if they are able to avoid circumstances or even people that may tempt them to use these substances. But food is different. Although some people are self-proclaimed food addicts, our physiological response to food is not comparable to our response to drugs. We simply can't give up food altogether. Not only is it everywhere but food is necessary for survival. It's not optional. Even if we wanted to, like that white bear or delicious chocolate cake, it's nearly impossible to stop thinking about food!

Short-Term Sacrifice Without the Reward

When most people start diets, they tend to think that they will change their eating behaviors temporarily; they will deprive themselves of "bad" foods for a short time until they lose their excess weight. Then, once they lose the weight, the diet will be over, and they can return to eating the foods they ate before. Maybe you've said things like "I am going on this diet until summer starts" or "I want to lose five pounds for my best friend's wedding." The focus tends to be on weight loss, with daily or regular "weigh-ins" providing encouraging (or discouraging) feedback about how you are doing on your diet. If all goes well, you avoid certain types or amounts of foods, and within days or weeks you hop on a scale to find that you weigh less. In this scenario, your sacrifice (eating less or different foods) is rewarded almost immediately (with a lower number on the scale). This, however, is not a strategic approach to weight loss and management for the long term. A successful diet should not be measured by how much you've lost after one week. This might make you feel great for a short time, but how are you going to feel when you just gain back all your weight after going off the diet at the end of the week? That is a shockingly unsuccessful diet!

Real, sustained weight loss requires thinking about weight management for the long term. And, by long term, I mean for the rest of your life. Weight loss isn't something that happens by the day or even by the week. Begin to think of weight loss as something that will gradually happen across a year. I know, I know—I can hear you grumbling now. A year sounds like a really long time to reach your ideal weight. But wouldn't you rather slowly lose weight over the next twelve months and keep it off for the rest of your life than lose twenty-five pounds in a month and gain it all back a few weeks later?

It is difficult for people to resist the immediate reward offered by rapid weight loss. People often (mistakenly) assume that losing weight will not only allow them to fit into a smaller pair of jeans but will immediately bring them confidence, happiness, and social rewards such as a new romantic partner or the admiration of their coworkers or family members. However, the emotional ups (following quick weight loss) and downs (following the inevitable regain of weight) actually leave people feeling worse about themselves in the long run.[8]

Dieting Makes You Feel Bad; Choose to Feel Good Instead

Losing weight feels good. It can be a first-rate confidence booster. In fact, in one study by the amazing diet researchers Janet Polivy and Peter Herman, people reported feeling better, thinner, and even *taller*, just for deciding to go on a diet (and they hadn't even lost any weight yet!).[9] However, jumping on a scale to find an upward weight fluctuation almost always leads dieters to feel despair. This is unfortunate because most of us will experience minor variations in our weight due to factors such as time of day, hormone fluctuations, and water retention.

Some individuals become so concerned about the numbers on the scale that what they "think" they weigh becomes more important than what they actually weigh. In one study, chronic dieters were weighed and were told either that they weighed five pounds more than they actually did or five pounds less.[10] As you can imagine, those who were told they weighed less than they actually did were pretty happy. But those that were told that they weighed more were upset. They weren't just upset about their weight; they felt bad about themselves in general and even experienced a decline in their self-esteem. It is important to remember that these individuals did not actually weigh more, they only *thought* they weighed more. In other words, the numbers on the scale were more important to their feelings and self-esteem than their actual body size. People who diet regularly (sometimes referred to as "restrained eaters") don't only experience low self-esteem but also believe that they are more unattractive, unhealthy, bad, weak, lazy, and out of control than did people who don't diet regularly. This is not exactly a great endorsement for dieting!

If I haven't convinced you yet that dieting isn't the best way to lose weight, try the following thought exercise (I promise, no more white bears or chocolate cake). Imagine that instead of reading these pages quietly to yourself, you're reading them to a crowd of two hundred people. How does that make you feel? Nervous? Anxious? While most people become nervous at the thought of public speaking—our hands get sweaty, our hearts beat a little faster, and we start to get that feeling of dread—chronic dieters tend to find this situation much more anxiety provoking than do people who don't regularly diet. But what does giving a speech have to do with dieting? Because chronic dieters are prone to anxiety and depression, they are less likely to cope with anxiety-causing situations (like public speaking).[11] This isn't to say that giving up dieting will make you love public speaking, but it may improve your psychological health in a variety of ways that may make you a happier, better-functioning person!

Dieting Leads to False Hope

It typically starts out well. We start a diet on Monday, of course, and we tend to feel good about ourselves for trying to change an element of our lives that we are not happy about: our weight. But, most of us dieters go through a cycle, sometimes referred to as "false hope syndrome," that tends to leave us feeling hopeful and good, only temporarily.[12]

Once the decision to go on a diet has been made, the next step is to actually take steps consistent with the diet of choice. Most of us can transition successfully from deciding to diet to implementing some behavior changes (e.g., eating less, cutting out certain foods) and will have some preliminary success on our diet. This leaves us feeling good and believing that weight loss is possible. However, we're inevitably challenged. We go to a party, we have to pick up a meal on the run, or we find ourselves in a circumstance that prohibits us from sticking to the plan, and we slip. This setback is pretty much unavoidable, as we all lead busy lives and few of us have personal chefs available to make the exact foods we want at the exact moment we want them.

Most of us who diet and experience a setback—whether it is due to a bad day or simply living a busy life—usually decide that the setback was our fault. "If only I'd practiced better will power at that party." "If only I'd packed a lunch and not gone through that drive-through." "If only I'd made some healthy food for the holidays and not relied on the traditional family favorites." Accepting responsibility for failure is usually commendable. But this is not necessarily true when it comes to dieting. It is likely—very likely—that your diet failed because of the diet itself, not because of you! If your diet does not allow for the irregularities in your schedule and the changing circumstances of your life, it is bound to fail. I know it, you know it, the CDC knows it, and the smartest research scientists who study dieting know it. Give yourself a break.

Deciding where the blame lies for dieting setbacks (and ultimate failure) is important. Most people place the blame on themselves: if they just try a little bit harder, they'll get it right the next time. So they embark on another attempt at dieting. Sometimes, it is the same diet that just failed them. Other times, it is a new diet plan. Regardless, the cycle begins: 1) decide to diet, 2) initial success on the diet, 3) inevitable failure on the diet, 4) deciding that failure was not inevitable, and 5) begin again.[13]

You know who is the most delighted that dieters fail but try again? The dieting industry. If dieting really worked, you'd only need to do it once. But the fact that it fails 98 percent of the time means big money for the diet industry. Just think about that number for a minute. Say I told you that a new car being manufactured broke down 98 percent of the time. Would you even think about buying that car? A company that produced such a lemon would see its profits vanish and quickly go out of business. However, in 2010, dieting industry profits were estimated to be $60.9 billion.[14] That's pretty exceptional, considering that we were in the midst of a global economic depression that year. This profit was not due to new customers, mind you. The diet industry relies on return customers—people who commit to dieting, are initially successful, inevitably "fail," and then recommit to try it all again.

Dieting Leads to Overeating

Let's say that you go on a diet and you decide that you will not be eating any sweets—candy, cookies, ice cream, cake, and the like. This decision has the unfortunate effect of turning sweets into "forbidden fruit," elevating these foods into objects of greater desire than if you hadn't told yourself you couldn't have them. So, what happens when you go to a birthday party and they are serving cake (and possibly cookies and ice cream as well)? You may be "good" on your diet and avoid these foods, or you may give in to temptation. Unfortunately, research indicates that if you do give in, you will eat more of these foods than you would have if you didn't label them as "forbidden." This tendency has been given a very scientific and descriptive name by dieting researchers: the "what-the-hell effect."[15]

If you are trying to diet and decide, "what the hell," and eat whatever you want, chances are you will end up eating more than you would if you had never tried to restrict yourself in the first place. This is exactly why some dieters will engage in binge eating (i.e., eating an extremely large amount in one sitting).[16] Essentially, they decide that once they have broken their diet, they might as well go crazy. Then, tomorrow (or, come Monday) they will recommit to being "good" and restrict themselves all over again. Sound familiar? Unfortunately, these episodes of overeating eliminate any benefit of successful dieting. One study that followed men and women for two years even found that those with a history of dieting weighed more at the end of the study than those without a history of dieting.[17] Given these findings, one has to wonder—what's the point?!

But if deciding not to eat certain foods leads you to overeat those very foods, how should you approach weight loss? Obviously, you can't eat cookies, cake, and ice cream every day without expecting to gain a few pounds. Plus, it's not healthy. Instead, you can begin to successfully lose weight and keep the weight off when you stop slapping the "forbidden" label on your favorite foods. Acknowledge that they bring you pleasure and joy and can be eaten in moderation. Many people are shocked to hear that I—a health psychologist who studies eating behaviors—eat dessert every night. But it's true. Pretty much every night, I indulge in dessert! Perhaps, a lot like you, I love sweets, and giving them up is not realistic for me. So, I enjoy a moderately sized portion of something sweet most evenings—sometimes it's ice cream; sometimes it's a few Hershey's Kisses; sometimes it's frozen yogurt. Not only do I enjoy the sweets, but I enjoy this ritual. I have found that when I have tried to eliminate this evening treat (e.g., after I had my children and hoped to lose my "baby weight"), I actually gained weight. Yes, you read that right—when I deprived myself of my evening sweet treat, I ended up gaining weight! Imagine that.

A recent study concurs with my advice to allow yourself to have some "forbidden foods" (should you desire them).[18] In this study, half of the participants were allowed a regular breakfast (300 calories), but the other half were given a large breakfast that contained something sweet (600 calories, with some calories coming from healthy foods and some coming from a donut, a piece of chocolate, or a biscuit). The first group, not allowed a morning sweet, initially lost weight but was unable to keep the weight off long-term. By contrast, the people in the "dessert for breakfast" group gradually but consistently lost weight after four months on this diet (in contrast, the other group started to regain weight loss after four months). These findings don't necessarily suggest that cake for breakfast is the fastest (or healthiest) route to weight loss. I can't advise having a heavy, sugar-laden breakfast on a regular basis. But what these findings demonstrate is that it is not necessary to restrict yourself entirely from favored foods. In other words, you can have your cake and lose weight, too!

In a rigorous analysis of 31 long-term diet studies, the majority of people regained all the lost weight, plus added more weight.

—**Traci Mann, professor of psychology, UCLA**

Dieting Can Lead to Weight Gain

So, you've now learned that you may be more likely to gain weight by cutting cake out of your diet than from eating it. And repeated attempts to diet lead to weight gain over time! There is a possible metabolic explanation for the link between dieting and weight gain (see page 33), but there is actually an easy-to-understand psychological explanation for what happens as well.

Let's say that you decide to go on a diet. Maybe the onset of summer (and the threat of wearing a swimsuit in public) is motivating you to try to lose ten pounds. So you decide to cut out dessert and snack foods. The first couple of days will go well. You feel virtuous for foregoing chips in the afternoons and ice cream after dinner. Then, on day 3 of your diet, you are stressed out and tired. You decide that a little ice cream after dinner will really cheer you up. What starts out as a reasonable half-cup portion quickly becomes a pint of Ben & Jerry's (the "what-the-hell" effect hits you). A couple of hours later, you feel miserable and guilty for ruining your new diet, and you vow to begin again the following day. Of course, the Ben & Jerry's binge erased any weight-loss benefits of the first couple of days of dieting. Further, your frustration with your lack of "will power" makes it hard to get back on track. You feel like you are bound to cheat on your diet again at some point. Days 4 and 5 of your diet may be a success, with hardly a single processed or high-fat food passing your lips. Then day 6 brings you to the weekend and a wonderful dinner out with your friends. A couple of cocktails into the outing and you decide to indulge in whatever foods you desire ("what the hell!"). This binge wipes out any benefits of the previous couple of days of restriction. It's about a week into your diet, and you haven't actually lost weight. In fact, if you were to weigh yourself the day after your dinner outing, you would likely weigh more than when you started. Obviously, this would feel far from encouraging.

This scenario represents a week in the life of many dieters. But it can also be used to understand many months in the lives of chronic dieters. Some will be successful for weeks on end. They'll cut out sweets or carbs or reduce their caloric intake. But these weeks of restriction leave them psychologically vulnerable to overeating when they finally do decide that they would like some cake, candy, or chips.[19] After all, most of us know that we can't live the rest of our life without indulging at some point. We seem inclined to diet as if we can entirely eliminate our favorite foods from our lives. Then, quitting or giving up on our diet leads to overindulgence in these foods we've deprived ourselves of for days, weeks, or months. Wouldn't it be better to just allow ourselves the foods we enjoy and not vacillate between dieting and overindulging? This is both a commonsense and totally radical idea to many long-term dieters.

JOLENE'S *Story*

In the last few years, I've been on more diets than I can keep track of. I did the low-carb and no-carb thing for a while. It worked and I lost weight, but I just couldn't go without bread for more than a few weeks. I liked the "flat belly diet," but that didn't last for more than a month. I invented my own diet that I called the "5 things diet." I tried to just eat five things, like one apple, one bagel, one yogurt, and two heaping servings of salad a day. Then I realized that those five servings just kept getting bigger (bagels can be huge!). I've come to realize that I'm good at losing weight, but I'm even better at gaining it back. After all of this dieting, I weigh more now than when I started. What a waste! All that suffering—for nothing!

None of this made any sense to me until I took Dr. Markey's Psychology of Eating class. Now I realize what a scam the dieting industry is. I also realize that weight loss can be a lot easier than most of us make it out to be. I've stopped "dieting" and have followed Dr. Markey's recommendations. I've actually lost weight! And, it's no big deal. I go out with my friends on the weekends, and I don't feel like I have to avoid eating certain foods. I eat three meals a day—and snacks. I pay attention to what I eat, but I'm learning not to be obsessed with food. I'm actually finding that I enjoy food a lot more, and my friends tell me that I seem happier. I only wish that I had understood the research about dieting a long time ago!

~Jolene, AGE TWENTY-TWO, STUDENT

Dieting Negatively Affects Your Metabolism

The word "metabolism" gets thrown around a lot today. Most of us have been led to believe that having a "fast" metabolism means that we can eat more than the average person without gaining weight. In contrast, having a "bad" or "slow" metabolism means that we're doomed to gain weight easily. However, this isn't entirely true. Our metabolism is not a fixed process that always operates the same way. Yes, we don't all have the same "speed" metabolism, but this isn't just because of genetics. Our genes and biology certainly affect our metabolism, but so do our eating habits.

Our bodies are designed to deal with the environment of our ancestors, not the modern world. In premodern times, shortages of food were common and excesses rare. Finding food took a great deal of energy, and the possibility of not having enough to eat at any given time was very likely. Thus, our metabolism was designed to function such that when we ate less (because food was scarce), our metabolism would slow down to protect us from starving. In other words, our bodies were designed to adjust to the food environment. Today, most of us have access to an abundance of food, and yet our metabolism still functions in the same premodern manner. This is partially why we seem to instinctually crave foods that are energy dense (e.g., full of fat) and likely to give us a quick boost of energy. Our premodern biology wants us to get full fast and stock up on foods that will keep us going for a long time—in case that next meal is a ways away.

However, when we eat less, our metabolism gradually slows down, and we gain weight more easily. This is one reason chronic dieters often complain that it is difficult to lose that last five pounds. As they lose weight, their bodies work against them, preparing for the possibility of starvation. "Yo-yo dieting" or patterns of chronic dieting—losing weight and gaining weight and losing weight again—are disruptions to our metabolism. Researchers have found that repeated metabolic disruptions make our bodies resistant to weight loss. Instead, they go into starvation mode![20] This is why chronic dieting has the potential to reduce our ability to metabolize food efficiently and effectively. This is also why diets that encourage extreme caloric restriction (even some of the time), such as the popular Fast Diet, may ultimately be counterproductive. The Fast Diet prescribes eating "regularly" for five days a week and fasting for two (women are advised to eat 500 calories and men 600 calories on a fasting day).[21] I can't imagine that the fasting days are much fun, but, more importantly, this behavior will not support healthy metabolic processes. In other words, in the long run, a "fast" diet only works to put the pounds back on . . . and fast!

So, how can you lose weight when your body is designed to keep your weight on to protect you from starving? The best way to keep your metabolism happy is with a gradual, long-term approach to changing your eating patterns. You have to give it time, and you have to be patient, but I've seen this work for my students, research participants, and even my own husband! This approach will not have negative consequences for your metabolism. On the contrary, avoiding food restriction and eating regular meals throughout the day may actually boost your metabolism. This is the most important difference between the majority of diets and my plan. It's not restrictive. I do not want you to feel hungry or deprived. I do not want your body to think you are starving and your metabolism to slow down. Rather, I want you to gradually develop healthy eating and activity patterns that will boost your mood, increase your fitness, and improve your health.

Both your metabolism and your waistline will thank you for these lifestyle changes.

Most people think of a diet as a project they take on to lose weight. They think that they will lose this weight and it will disappear and never return to them. If this was how our bodies worked, then diets like the Fast Diet that prescribe dramatic food restriction would work. But the problem is our bodies and our metabolism doesn't work this way. A comparison can be made between the way we attempt to achieve our ideal weight and how we obtain our desired temperature in our home. My husband and I always disagree on the ideal temperature. Many mornings he turns the thermostat way down to make our house colder. At a later point, I then turn the thermostat way up. The problem is, neither of us is really happy with this situation. The temperature in our home swings up and down over the course of the day. Both our marriage and our electric bill would be better off if we simply worked on a system where we gradually adjusted the thermostat to a temperature that made us both happy. An analogous dynamic happens with our weight. If we "turn down" the amount or types (e.g., high fat, calorie dense) of food we put into our body, our weight will go down. But, when we start to feed ourselves more, our weight will go back up. Our weight then starts to yo-yo up and down as we adjust our "internal thermostats." In other words, we need to reset our weight thermostats to a place where we plan to stay and find a way to keep ourselves at this new weight. We do this by gradually working toward a relatively healthy, maintainable way of eating. We need to find what works for us. The goal isn't to be constantly fiddling with our weight thermostats but to find a body weight (and the related amount and way we eat) that keeps us healthy and feeling good.

A diet is a plan, generally hopeless, for reducing your weight, which tests your will power but does little for your waistline.

—Herbert B. Prochnow, banking executive and author

Weight Loss That Works

Usually, when I explain the information in this chapter to my students, at least half of them tell me that they find this incredibly depressing. Diets don't work!? Then what are we supposed to do? The more I've studied these issues, the more I actually find this conclusion inspiring. Really! I mean, who actually wants to go on a diet anyway? It's actually pretty thrilling and even freeing to realize that dieting is a bad idea and there is a better way—an approach that is supported by science!

I do understand why people find the idea of going on a diet appealing, though. The majority of diet plans available offer very specific prescriptions for weight loss in very precise amounts of time. I understand why these specifics may be reassuring to people. We make countless food choices each day (for ourselves and other people), and there is something potentially easier about just having someone else make those choices for us. But, hopefully, this chapter has convinced you that these sorts of plans don't work. Instead, a personalized, gradual, health-conscious approach to weight management is what you need. In the upcoming chapters, I'll provide guidelines for getting your new approach to eating underway. This approach will give you a lot of flexibility to make the basic premise of this book work for you. So, let go of the old you who relied on diets and embark on a new you—a happier, thinner, and, most importantly, healthier you!

- Diets aren't fun and they don't work.
- Diets are more likely to lead to weight gain than weight loss.
- What the heck *can* you do? Be smart. Take a long-term, healthy approach.

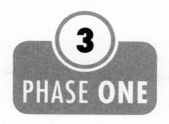

Honestly Weigh In

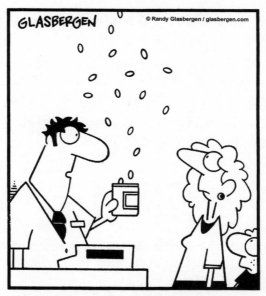

"Take a few capsules each morning before
you weigh yourself. They're filled
with helium."

Great results cannot be achieved at once; and we
must be satisfied to advance in life as we walk, step
by step.

Samuel Smiles, author and government reformer

f you are anything like me, when you want something, you want it *now*. Patience is not my greatest virtue! This is especially true when it comes to something I really care about. And, many of us care about our weight. We want to be thinner—yesterday. However, having patience when it comes to weight loss will pay off in the future. One of my students described her feelings about this nicely this past semester: "There are easier ways to actually lose weight and keep it off! Making a healthy lifestyle change and sticking to it will be beneficial to me. Basically, because Dr. Markey crushed my hopes about get-slim-quick diets, I've been forced to find the better way to make a change. I know it will save me money, time, tears, and pounds." The "better way" that she is referring to is the approach that starts with Phase 1: honestly weigh in. I appreciate why you may be reluctant to give up on the hope you once had of losing twenty-one pounds in twenty-one days (or whatever get-slim-quick approach you've favored), but remember all that ever was, was a fantasy; it is not a realistic way to lose weight and keep it off.

Get Started Today

Don't wait until Monday. Don't wait until January 1 or bathing-suit season. Start today! But, before you get started, it's important that you recognize that there is no "one-size-fits-all" approach to healthy weight loss and management. You need to understand your eating patterns and preferences, why and when you do or don't exercise (although I'll delve into exercise in more detail in Chapter 6), and how all of this makes you feel. It might feel "easier" to just be given a specific plan; I know you have enough other stuff to worry about. However, I also know that that won't work; *you* need to do some of the work! The best place to start is by monitoring what you eat and when you exercise over the course of an average week. Being honest with yourself and really getting to know your habits is incredibly important. We all maintain habits that are potentially embarrassing, whether it is our total lack of exercise or our ten-

In this chapter you will learn . . .

- How to take inventory of your current height, weight, and body mass index
- How to set realistic fitness and weight loss goals
- Tips for recording your typical daily food intake and physical activity

dency to eat breakfast in the car each morning. One of the best-kept secrets of healthy weight loss and management is to come to terms with the habits that don't facilitate health and gradually change them. Today is as good as any day to begin to become more aware of the good and bad elements of your daily eating and exercise behaviors.

Your body is the baggage you must carry through life. The more excess the baggage, the shorter the trip.
—Arnold H. Glasgow, businessman and humorist

Your Initial Weigh-In

First things first: find an accurate medical scale to assess your weight. No need to go out and purchase a fancy one because after this initial weigh-in, you will not be using it much. If you don't own a scale that you're confident is accurate, borrow a friend's scale, or weigh yourself at the gym or your doctor's office. You want to pick a time of day (I recommend the morning) and circumstances (e.g., with or without clothes) that you can replicate for the occasional weigh-in. It's typical for everyone to experience minor weight fluctuations (a few pounds) from day to day and even at different times of the day, so you want to be as consistent as possible. Don't weigh yourself with clothes and a heavy jacket today and then in your birthday suit a week from now. Otherwise, that two-pound loss recorded on the scale will not be true weight loss.

Assessing your weight by itself is not that useful in terms of understanding your health. So you also need to measure your height. Many of us think we know how tall we are, but this perception of our height is not necessarily accurate, so it is worth taking a few minutes to do this. (My driver's license says that I am 5'6", but I'm at least an inch shorter. I never intended to lie—I was just being optimistic when I acquired my license at sixteen, and I've never changed it!) To get an accurate measurement, ask a friend to help you with a tape measure. Next, you'll use these measurements to calculate your body mass index, or BMI.

Calculating Your Body Mass Index

Your body mass index is a metric of weight status that takes into account both your height and your weight. Calculate your BMI by dividing your weight in pounds by your height in inches squared, and then multiply this number by 703.

BMI Formula: weight (lb) / [height (in)]^2 x 703
Example: Weight = 140 lbs, Height = 5'4" (64")
Calculation: $[140 \div (64)^2] \times 703 = 24.03$

If you don't have a calculator handy, you can use the BMI calculator on the CDC's web page (all you have to do is enter your weight and height): http://www.cdc.gov/healthyweight/assessing/bmi/adult_bmi/english_bmi_calculator/bmi_calculator.html.

Once you've figured out your BMI, you can get a sense of how healthy your weight status is by referencing the table below. It is important to understand that BMI is a rough, but important, indicator of a person's health.[1] As I'll describe later, all sorts of health issues, ranging from cancer risk to diabetes, are affected by what we eat and our weight status. Individuals who fall in the overweight and obese category are at increased risk of health problems. However, BMI is *not* an indicator of attractiveness. In fact, it is quite possible that you may find yourself in the healthy weight category and still desire weight loss. Most of the models and celebrities that we are inclined to want to physically resemble likely find themselves in the underweight category. This does *not* mean that the average person should aim to be underweight. Being underweight confers health risks including anemia, nutrient deficiencies, osteoporosis, cardiovascular irregularities, vulnerability to infection and disease, delayed wound healing, infertility and pregnancy complications (for women), lack of energy, and even depression.[2] So, in thinking about your weight loss or weight maintenance goals, it is important to stay within a "healthy" weight range.

BMI	WEIGHT CATEGORY
Below 18.5	Underweight
18.5 – 24.9	Healthy
25.0 – 29.9	Overweight
30.0 and Above	Obese

The tables below provides examples of weight ranges, BMI ranges, and weight category for two different heights.

EXAMPLE HEIGHT	WEIGHT RANGE	BMI	WEIGHT CATEGORY
5'5"	111 lbs or less	Below 18.5	Underweight
5'5"	112 to 149 lbs	18.5 – 24.9	Healthy
5'5"	150 to 180 lbs	25.0 – 29.9	Overweight
5'5"	181 lbs or more	30.0 or higher	Obese

EXAMPLE HEIGHT	WEIGHT RANGE	BMI	WEIGHT CATEGORY
6'0"	136 lbs or less	Below 18.5	Underweight
6'0"	137 to 183 lbs	18.5 – 24.9	Healthy
6'0"	184 to 220 lbs	25.0 – 29.9	Overweight
6'0"	221 lbs or more	30.0 or higher	Obese

When you look at these tables, you may be surprised at the wide range of weight statuses that are considered normal and healthy. It is important that we all think about what is a healthy and comfortable weight range for ourselves within this normal weight range. As opposed to focusing on a single number for our ideal weight, it is much healthier to think about a five- or ten-pound range that we want to aim to stay within. We will not weigh the exact same amount each and every day, no matter how hard we try. Everything from the holidays to our hormones has the potential to cause our weight to fluctuate a little bit. If you can accept this, you will begin to feel less tortured by the scale. And, believe me, what a relief this is!

Understanding BMI

You may find it surprising that men and women do not have different weight categories for BMI. Usually, men are larger and weigh more than women. But, this is because men are typically taller than women. In spite of this, the association between BMI and percentage of body fat is fairly strong.[3] Many professional athletes have high BMIs because they have more muscle mass relative to body fat, so they tend to be in good physical shape despite their elevated numbers. However, for you and me (i.e., individuals who are not professional athletes), a high BMI is *almost* always an indicator of serious health risk.

At different times in my life, I have changed my exercise regimen and found that I *gained* weight, not lost it. I have been comforted by the popular conception that "muscle weighs more than fat," and my increased exercise must be making me more muscular, but not necessarily larger. However, it turns out that this is a cop-out, both in terms of oversimplifying the relation between exercise and body composition and in terms of understanding BMI. A pound is a pound. Yes, a pound of fat may look less appealing than a pound of muscle on a person's body. But most of us who gain weight are not gaining it in muscle. Gaining muscle mass is difficult to do and requires regular, arduous exercise across many months, if not years. Gaining fat is relatively easy to do and can happen in weeks. It is one of the many things about life that is unfair. All of this is to say that most of us cannot blame a high BMI on muscle mass. If you are an athlete or an extremely athletic person who spends several hours a day in the gym, you might not need to worry about your high BMI. The rest of us most likely need to lose weight when our weight status falls in the overweight or obese categories.

More Than BMI

Although I (and many others[4]) endorse the use of BMI as a rough metric of weight and health status, it would be irresponsible of me not to mention that all of us have family histories, psychological factors, experiences, and circumstances that contribute to our health.

BMI is unquestionably an imperfect measure of weight status, but more precise measures are typically costly, complicated, and less reliable (e.g., measuring the percentage body fat). However, one relatively easy assessment that helps to gauge our overall health is waist circumference. People who carry their weight around their waist (sometimes referred to as having an "apple shape") as opposed to people who carry their weight around their hips (sometimes referred to as having a "pear shape") tend to be at higher risk for health problems including type 2 diabetes and heart disease. So, before beginning any attempt at weight loss, you may want to measure your waist as well. To do this, breathe out and place a tape measure around your middle. You should measure your waist above your hipbones. If you are a woman, your risk of health problems increases when your waist is thirty-five inches or greater. If you are a man, your risk of health problems increases when your waist is forty inches or greater.[5]

Finally, before diving in to any weight loss plan, you may want to consider a visit to your primary care physician (PCP) to assess any vulnerability you may have to cardiovascular disease, diabetes, elevated blood pressure, or cancer. Although all adults should have regular well visits with their PCP, usually we go only when we think we need a prescription for something. Use this as an excuse to at least have your blood pressure checked and blood work done to check your cholesterol levels. Consider going back to your PCP next year and have these assessments done again once you've lost weight—you will be amazed at how your health will benefit from following the recommendations in this book!

Setting Goals

Now that you have taken inventory of your current weight status and understand how you're measuring up, so to speak, it is time to set some goals for yourself. If you are maintaining a healthy, normal weight, you really shouldn't be setting a goal to lose fifty pounds, or you risk succumbing to health problems associated with being underweight (e.g., osteoporosis, cardiovascular irregularities, susceptibility to infection, infertility, etc.). If you are maintaining a healthy weight status but want to lose a significant amount of weight, evaluate your motives for weight loss carefully. It may make sense to talk with a counselor or nutritionist if you feel distraught about your weight but are maintaining a healthy weight by medical standards. Being overly concerned about your weight while maintaining a healthy weight can be indicative of an eating disorder or may place you at risk for developing one. Eating disorders are very serious medical conditions that take an extraordinary toll on individuals' mental and physical health and well-being. If you think you may be at risk, I strongly urge you to seek professional help immediately. (If you aren't sure where to start, the National Eating Disorder Association's web page, NationalEatingDisorders.org, includes support and referral information.)

It is important to remember that the advice I offer in this book is not only evidence based but applicable to all people interested in losing weight or maintaining a healthy weight. Whether you want to lose five pounds or fifty, the steps you take to achieve your weight goals are essentially the same, with improved health (not just improved appearance) being your ultimate outcome. However, if, by BMI standards, you currently fall into the overweight or obese category, research suggests that your health is likely to substantially benefit from losing just 10 percent of your body weight.[6] So, for example, if you are a 5'5" tall woman who weighs two hundred pounds, losing twenty pounds will significantly improve your health. You may want to lose much more than twenty pounds, but it is important to recognize that this is a good initial goal. Start small—you can create more ambitious goals later, but set achievable goals now. Remember, it is better to lose five pounds *permanently* than it is to lose twenty-five pounds for three months only to gain it (and maybe a few more) back three months later. You can use my recommendations to continually revise your goals, but it is important that each goal you set is realistic.

Even if you have a vacation booked or a high school reunion on the horizon, it's important that you don't give yourself strict time limits or set goals of losing excessive amounts of weight when you begin this plan. Remember, you are going to keep the weight off for the rest of your life—you have time. You should have a range of weight that you'd like to lose, such as, "I'd like to lose four to seven pounds this month" or "I'd like to lose twenty to twenty-five pounds in the next six months." Depending on your current weight and eating and activity patterns, it is unlikely that you can healthily lose more than one to two pounds per week and maintain that weight loss. If you are significantly overweight, weigh loss may be a bit faster (two to three pounds per week), but beware of unrealistic expectations. I appreciate that it may not be very motivating to set the goal of losing one pound during a week and then step on the scale at the end of that week to find that you lost . . . one pound. This is why you need to think long-term. Set a goal for the next month (lose five pounds), the next six months (lose twenty pounds total), and the next year (lose thirty pounds total). Or, consider setting a goal for this month (lose three pounds) and then evaluate how this month goes for you before setting a goal for the next month.

Realistic goals for weight loss are important for many reasons. Of course, it is hard to quantify what is realistic for any given person, but obviously losing ten pounds in one day or even one week is not realistic for anyone. Remember, one of the many reasons that most diets ultimately fail is that we often are unrealistic about how fast and how easy it will be to lose weight. We also tend to be unrealistic about how our lives will change once we lose weight.[7] In one study, people reported believing that losing weight would make them more likely to win the lottery.[8] This is a fabulous notion, but unfortunately you cannot begin a weight-loss plan believing that losing weight will automatically lead you to enjoy professional and personal success. Weight loss has many advantages, but believing it will make you happier, wealthier, and taller (really, people have reported expecting to grow taller!) only leads to disappointment.

Setting realistic, incremental goals is psychologically important when you are trying to lose weight. And not being overly rigid about these goals is critical. To permanently lose weight, you can't beat yourself up over every Hershey's Kiss that passes your lips; you need to be flexible and understanding with yourself. You can't punish yourself if you don't achieve your goals as quickly as you'd like. I remember feeling somewhat disappointed when I gradually (following the advice I offer in this book) lost the weight I had gained while pregnant with my first child. It felt like such an accomplishment to put my old jeans back on. No one but me seemed to notice when that last five pounds was lost (and I certainly wasn't any wealthier). This was one of the many times I came to realize that we care about our *exact* weight a lot more than other people care about our exact weight. We may guard what we weigh as if it is a national secret (even more than we guard our age!), but other people are not as judgmental of us as we are of ourselves.

Always keep in mind that this is not about achieving short-term weight loss; you are changing your eating and activity patterns for the rest of your life. Celebrate your successes, no matter how small they are. Maybe you lost one or two pounds this month. This is fantastic! Treat yourself to an extra round of golf or a pedicure as a reward. It may seem counterintuitive to award such "small" accomplishments, but being less rigid and less punishing of yourself will actually help you to achieve your goal of permanent weight loss.

Start to Record and Record Everything

Now that you have assessed your weight status and started to think about your achievable short- and long-term weight goals, it is time to begin to record and get a better understanding of how much you eat, when you eat, what you eat, and your general level of physical activity. It is important for you to know up front that you will be recording your food and activities for only about a week. So although it may be challenging to stick with this, it only needs to be for seven days. You can do this with the food diary sheet on the next page that I have asked participants in my research to use to record their eating and activity patterns. You may want to photocopy this page (or download it from www.Smart PeopleDontDiet.com). Or, you may want to type out your eating and activity patterns in a Word document. Others have found that it is easier to use their smartphone along with various apps available for these devices (see some suggestions that are provided later in this chapter). Every beverage and food item should be accounted for (even water). Calorie count, however, is not required, and I'll explain why later. Walking half a mile to pick your kids up from school counts as physical activity (although I'd say that walking up the stairs in your house does not unless you have a lot of stairs or make a point of going up and down them many times). The most important thing is to be very thorough and take note of the time of day and everything you ate or drank with as much

|||||||||||||||||||||||||||||||||||||||||||||||||||||||||||||||||||||||||||||||||||||||||||||||||||||||||||||||

Food Diary

TIME	FOOD/DRINKS CONSUMED/ PHYSICAL ACTIVITIES	REFLECTION/MOOD
6am		
7am		
8am		
9am		
10am		
11am		
12pm		
1pm		
2pm		
3pm		
4pm		
5pm		
6pm		
7pm		
8pm		
9pm		
10pm		
11pm		
12midnight		
1am		

detail as possible. Record whatever physical activity you participated in, and reflect on how you felt (both physically and mentally) about your eating, drinking, and activity.

When I ask my students or participants in my research to record what they eat, they always start off enthusiastically. However, after a couple of days they start to complain that it gets hard to remember to record all of this. Some admit feeling bad when they see everything they've eaten laid out in front of them. This shouldn't be an exercise that evokes negative feelings. Consider this a mission to get to know yourself better, and make a plan about the things you can do to remember to keep recording. Set your alarm on your smartphone to go off around mealtime as a cue to record. Tell the people that you eat with what you are doing and ask them to help you remember (better yet, ask them to record their own eating and activity behaviors so that you can remind each other!). I recommend recording throughout the day, as we tend to "forget" foods (usually unhealthy foods) if we wait. Remember, you are only doing this for a week, but it is a crucial step toward modifying your eating behaviors and managing your weight. You have to take this seriously if you are committed to losing weight. Record everything. Even those few chips that you just mindlessly snacked on—write it down.

What Technology Has to Offer

Although I suggest recording anything and everything you eat and all sorts of activities that you participate in, I realize that this can be burdensome and difficult at times. Fortunately, you do not need to have a piece of paper with you at all times anymore to do this effectively. New apps, web pages, and devices to monitor our eating and fitness behaviors are being designed all the time; by the time I finish writing this paragraph, it is likely that another device or app will be created. A recent report suggests that seven out of ten adults in the United States monitor their weight, diet, exercise, or some other aspect of their health.[9] Most don't use technology, but there is speculation that it will be increasingly helpful as these new devices and apps are refined to make them increasingly user friendly. Recently, an electronic fork (somewhat ironically, I think, named, HAPIfork) was created that can help you monitor what you eat. When you start to eat too fast, it vibrates.[10] Although I'm not convinced that this particular device will prove helpful with your efforts to manage your weight, other technology-based programs and apps may prove extremely helpful. The good thing is that you don't need to spend a lot of time or money selecting an app or other device; I don't advise that you continue to monitor your food intake forever. Once you adopt some healthy habits and get the hang of my approach, it is healthy to lay off the recording. Nothing ruins eating more than feeling like it is an endless homework assignment!

As you can see from these descriptions, some people have been able to incorporate technology into their weight loss strategy, whereas others find it more difficult to balance technology with their daily life. Different technology features appeal to different people, so take the following recommendations with a grain of salt, and play around with a few until you find the one that feels the most helpful. If none of this is for you, that's okay, too!

> **Here's what some users I surveyed had to say about their ventures into technology-assisted, nondieting weight management:**
>
> I use the Lose It! app and I really like it. It made me realize how quickly a little of this and a little of that can add up and that the difference between gaining and maintaining (or losing) is awareness, for me at least. It also made me realize that it doesn't need to be about major deprivation; slow and steady can do wonders. **~Sara, age thirty-six**
>
> My partner hates when I enter my Weight Watchers points at the dinner table. **~Holly, age thirty-two**
>
> My Fitbit is an incredible tool that keeps me accountable daily for my calories (burned and eaten), weight, and activity. It automatically syncs to my computer and keeps me motivated to achieve my personal goals by providing online tools that chart activity, weight and calories over time. I love it! **~Susan, age fifty-five**

SmartenFit. As I did research for this section of the book, I came to realize that there were many health, diet, and fitness apps available, but none embodied the philosophy of this book or provided all the features that I thought were necessary to do what I advise. Thus, SmartenFit was born! In collaboration with two women with PhDs and complementary expertise in health, diet, social psychology, user experience, and technology use, I designed SmartenFit to include features that allow you to calculate and track your BMI, keep a food diary (using photos and text), set healthy (realistic and achievable) goals, generate healthy alternatives to the foods we all love, and think about weight loss and management as an important long-term investment in your health. The app also features health-related articles, motivational words, and tips vetted by me and other researchers I trust. The purpose of the app is to provide a simple and user-friendly way to employ the recommendations in this book to promote moderation and general record keeping (not every little thing needs to be recorded, not every little calorie counted) for long-term sustainable lifestyle change.

> **Pro:** This app is extremely user friendly, intended to assist long-term weight management, and designed to help you do everything recommended in this book. You can get more information at www .SmartenFit.com or scan the QR code on the back cover.
>
> **Con:** Just like this book, if you are interested in a fad or get-slim-quick scheme, you won't find it here. Sorry.

MyFitnessPal. This is a free app for the iPhone and can be used online at www.myfitnesspal.com. It has consistently been among the top-rated apps since its release.[11] MyFitnessPal allows you to calculate eating and fitness goals based on your current height and weight and your goal weight. It allows you to enter information about the exercise that you do, and it turns this information into calories burned. However, the feature that it is best known for is its extensive database of food items to help you track your food intake, including particular brands of foods, restaurant meals, and even recipes. Further, it allows you to enter a new food to the database should you be able to find something to eat that is not among the million or more food items already included.

Pro: Users of this app find it to be easy and fast to use, taking just minutes to log an entire day's worth of information.

Con: It has more bells and whistles than you need and may promote more specific recording than you want.

Lose It! This app is also free and has many of the positive features of MyFitnessPal and connects to a website, www.LoseIt.com. This app will take the calories burned exercising and apply them to the number you have designated for your calorie intake (i.e., the more you exercise, the more you can eat in a day without going over your limit). Although this is a fun feature, I can't recommend excessive exercise in the name of overeating. Moderation in both exercise and eating is a safer bet over the long term. This app will also scan bar codes of products to determine nutritional information.

Pro: Like MyFitnessPal, it is rated as very easy to use by consumers.

Con: All of this recording and the detailed features can start to feel like a never-ending school project.

Weight Watchers. The Weight Watchers app is another free option, but connecting to the online community or really joining Weight Watchers is not free (www.WeightWatchers.com). Weight Watchers' prescriptions for weight management are similar to many of the prescriptions offered in this book and focus on the adoption of healthy, long-term eating and activity habits. However, Weight Watchers utilizes a point system, as opposed to a recording of calories, fat, carbs, protein, or fiber. So, when consumers enter food items, their "point value" is determined by the app, and users are advised to consume a particular number of points per day (based on their height, weight, and weight loss goals).

Pro: The point system is unique and may make keeping track of what is eaten easier.

Con: I don't prescribe keeping track of what you eat forever, and if you have ever spent time around someone on the Weight Watchers plan, you know how irritating it is to hear about the point values attributed to specific foods.

Fitbit. A Fitbit (approximately $100) is a device that you wear (or stick in your pocket) that measures your heart rate, steps, calories, and can even tell you when you fall asleep and how many times you wake up. Its partner website is www.FitBit.com. The Fitbit can tell you how much you have exercised, or calories burned, across the day without you actually entering any information into the device (you have it on you). Fitbit has also developed a similar, bracelet-like device (see http://www.fitbit .com/flex) that not only tracks activity and sleep patterns but also allows you to determine your progress toward daily goals based on lights illuminated on the device.

Pro: Users love that it is small and powerful and has wireless syncing capabilities.

Con: Aside from the price tag, I have heard complaints about the device being unreliable when exposed to any moisture, which is a problem if you wear this while exercising and you break a sweat.

Pro *and* Con: The Fitbit's constant tracking of your progress may prove motivating. However, I do think there are real drawbacks to knowing *this* much. I think that the Fitbit may be fun to use initially, but is unlikely to support a long-term approach to healthy weight management. After all, do you actually want to know exactly how many calories you have consumed and burned every day for the rest of your life?

Nike Fuelband. Nike's Fuelband (and updated Nike+ Fuelband SE) is similar to the Fitbit in many ways (http://www.nike.com/us/en_us/lp /nikeplus-fuelband; cost approximately $150). The Fuelband is actually a band that you wear around your wrist. It is made to look athletic and a bit futuristic. As you move, the device keeps track of your activity. It also tells the time, if you are one of those folks who don't rely on your cell phone as your clock.

> **Pro:** The Fuelband allows you to set daily activity goals, and a color-coded system on the band lets you know how well you are progressing toward them. It syncs with your smartphone and computer and allows you to connect with your friends.
>
> **Con:** Consumers complain about the band being uncomfortable and moving around (although it is water resistant), and my concerns about it are generally the same as my concerns with the Fitbit: this may be a bit TMI for most people and may foster compulsive goal-setting and activity levels that are not maintainable across the long haul.

UP band. Similar to Fitbit and the Nike Fuelband, the UP band (and the newer UP24; https://jawbone.com/up; cost approximately $150) claims to track how you "sleep, move, and eat—then, helps you use that information to feel your best."

> **Pro:** This waterproof device communicates wirelessly with your smartphone and looks cooler than some of the other devices (at least I think so). You pay for style, but if it makes becoming health conscious more fun, then it is a minor financial investment that may pay for itself over time.
>
> **Con:** If you plan to follow my advice to monitor your habits for a week at a time only periodically, then the gizmos provided by all of these devices and bands may prove to be an unnecessary expense. Further, you may be able to get a simpler app, like SmartenFit, that gives you the information that you really need.

Runkeeper and MapMyRun. If you want a computer-based but somewhat simpler approach to tracking fitness goals, you may want to check out www.Runkeeper.com or www.MapMyRun.com and their corresponding apps. These free apps and web programs allow you to keep track of and map (as their names suggest) runs, walks, and outdoor fitness activities. They also allow for tracking other activities as diverse as ice skating and skiing. My friends and I who run together typically use these apps, especially when we are training for a race.

> **Pro:** They aren't super fancy, but you can chart your progress in achieving fitness goals, determine calories burned during exercise, share information with friends, and it is fun to log on to the web page and see yourself gradually getting in better shape.
>
> **Con:** Like any of these apps, ongoing recording may prompt more attention to numbers (e.g., calories consumed, calories burned, miles ran) than is really necessary.

In Chapter 6, I'll discuss physical activity as a part of long-term weight management and health in greater detail. For now, it is important to remember that you are merely recording what you *usually* do. If you don't usually exercise, you have nothing to record, and that's okay. If you prefer to avoid these gizmos and web pages and just write down what you eat and when you exercise in a journal of some sort, that is okay, too. The technology is always advancing, and new apps, web pages, and devices are available each day.

You don't have to be great to start, but you have to start to be great.

— Zig Ziglar

Honesty Is the Best Dieting Policy

Once you start to honestly record your eating habits and physical activities, it may be tempting to dramatically change what you eat. Resist. Eventually, I will encourage you to change what you eat—bite by bite—but not yet. Right now, I just want you to begin to understand how you *typically* eat and the extent to which you typically exercise. For the time being, observe what you do throughout the course of a typical week. Do your best to include notes about how you felt at different points in the day. Did eating that oatmeal for breakfast make you feel ready to take on the day? Did having McDonald's for dinner make you feel guilty? Did running three miles after work make you feel relaxed? Try to be totally honest with yourself. Honesty is the best approach to long-term weight loss and management.

To give you an idea of what a typical food diary looks like, read through Julie and Lilly's (see pages 58–59). They were average-weight students in my Psychology of Eating class who were in their early twenties. They were interested in losing about five pounds (aren't we all?) but were far from obsessed with their weight. Take notice of the amount of detail included regarding the portion sizes they consumed. You do not need to start to measure and weigh your food while you record what you eat during this first week. It is okay to approximate portion sizes, but if you are unsure of how to do this, then get out a measuring cup or pay attention to serving-size information on food labels. Lilly's food diary does not include a lot of information about specific portion sizes, and yet you can get a pretty good idea of what she ate on this particular Thursday and Friday. Importantly, when I ask people to record what they eat and reflect on this, I ask them to always keep records from weekdays and weekends to compare. Likewise, you should also be sure that you keep good records for at least a few weekdays and weekend days. For a variety of reasons, our eating habits tend to be somewhat different on the weekdays and weekends, and it is important to become aware of these variations. Notice how Julie made brief notes about her mood throughout the day. These do not need to be extensive, but they can prove helpful. For example, maybe every time you exercise you feel relaxed, and every time you eat chips you feel guilty. This will help you understand the kinds of changes in your regular patterns of behavior that are likely to make you feel better—and become healthier!

We're All Cheaters at Some Point

After reading Julie and Lilly's food diaries, you might start to realize that it can be hard to accurately and honestly report your food and physical activity. There are many, many ways you can cheat during this record-keeping phase. We are all vulnerable to cheating, myself included. Here are some of the ways that I find myself cheating when I embark on a stint of keeping track of my diet and exercise (yes, I still do this; you'll understand why after you read Chapter 8).

- If I'm eating my kids' leftovers I tend to "forget" to count or record it (after all, the food would go to waste if I didn't eat it, so eating it is the right thing to do).
- If I'm tasting food while I prepare it, I often don't record it. Of course, a quick lick of a sauce is not a big deal and fine to forget. But, when you have a spoon out and you are finishing off a bowl of chocolate chip cookie dough, that definitely counts.
- Eating while standing up tends to get overlooked. It's not my fault I'm a busy mom.
- Calories you drink can't be as bad for you as calories you eat—right? And, alcohol can't have *that* many calories in it.
- A few gummy bears are ignored when it comes time to record (never mind that I rarely really eat only a few and that there's up to 10 calories in each one; overall, not a good snack food).
- Condiments don't count. And butter is a condiment—right?

(*continues on page 60*)

|||||||||||||||||||||||||||||||||||||||||||||||||||||||||||||||||||||||||||||||||||||||||||||||||||||||||||||

Julie's Food Diary, age twenty-two

TIME	FOOD/DRINKS CONSUMED/ PHYSICAL ACTIVITIES	REFLECTION/MOOD
6am		
7am	Coffee w/ 2 splenda and ¼ cup of half and half Oatmeal (package; 180 cal)	Fine, tired
8am		
9am	Banana	More awake, fine
10am		
11am		
12pm	Ham sandwich (2 pieces of wheat bread, 2 slices of ham, mustard, lettuce); water	Good
1pm		
2pm	Bag of Doritos chips (cool ranch flavor); diet coke	Guilty about chips, but they tasted good
3pm	Walked for 30 minutes on treadmill	Great while walking; relaxed
4pm	Apple dipped in peanut butter (1 tablespoon); water	Good
5pm		
6pm	2 cups pasta w/ pesto sauce. 1 small grilled chicken breast (about 5 in by 4 in). 1 cup of carrots. 1 glass white wine.	Fine
7pm		
8pm		
9pm	Ben and Jerry's ice cream, chocolate chip cookie dough flavor (1 cup)	Tired
10pm		
11pm		
12midnight		
1am		

General Reflection   *How do you feel about what you ate and the physical activity that you did/did not participate in?*

This was a pretty typical day of eating and activity for me. I would have liked to have had more time to exercise, but I couldn't squeeze anything else in. I ate some "bad" foods (chips, ice cream), but I enjoyed them and did not feel like making a different or better choice.

||||||||||||||||||||||||||||||||||||||||||||||||||||||||||||||||||||||||||||||||||||||||||||||||||||||||||||||||

Lilly's Food Diary, age twenty-five

THURSDAY

Breakfast
-One cup English Breakfast tea with 1 packet Sugar in the Raw
-One medium banana
-One piece whole wheat toast with 1 tablespoon Nutella hazelnut spread
-One medium hot Dunkin' Donuts coffee, cream, and Splenda

Lunch
-Chicken tenders, breaded and fried (2)
-Small to medium serving French fries (no larger than McDonald's medium size)
-Ketchup for dipping
-BBQ sauce for dipping
-22 oz water

Dinner
-Four small onion rings with thousand island dressing for dipping
-One salad, with light shredded cheese, oil, and vinegar
-Two slices whole wheat bread with butter (light)
-1/2 chicken breast with sautéed mushrooms (in red wine sauce)
-One portabella mushroom cap with grated parmesan cheese
-Steamed broccoli, squash, carrots, sugar snap peas, and cauliflower (Salt and pepper to taste)
-Water with lemon (2 glasses)

Dessert
-One serving Tastykake coffee cakes (2 cakes)
-One cup Black Tiger Extra Bold coffee, 1 packet Sugar in the Raw, 2 tablespoons half and half

FRIDAY

Breakfast
-Two buttermilk waffles with margarine (one teaspoon) and lite syrup (two tablespoons)
-One cup English Breakfast tea with 1 packet Sugar in the Raw

Lunch
-One slice cheese pizza (medium slice)
-22 oz water

Snack
-Small Clementine (2)

Dinner
-Sautéed ham (spiral cut) and potatoes (fresh from my uncle's farm)
-Roasted red onions, green peppers, red peppers, and yellow squash
-Salt and pepper to taste
-22 oz water
-1 glass milk (1 percent fat)

Dessert
-Half of a small sized bag of movie theater popcorn, butter added
-2 glasses water

- Running after my kids counts as exercise. Although I found a web page suggesting that this may lead to burning about 100 calories in thirty minutes, when I'm honest with myself I know that this is more mentally than physically taxing. There are better ways to exercise.

Any of these sound familiar? Maybe you tell yourself similar tales? Even those of us invested in eating well are not always as honest with ourselves as we need to be. It is easy to overlook, or consciously ignore, a few hundred calories per day. However, if we recognize these sorts of habits and improve upon them, this may be all we need to do to start losing weight. This is exactly why you need to record *everything.* A lot of the things we may be apt to overlook when we keep our food diaries are the exact same things we should be looking to change in our diet!

So, let's assume Julie and Lilly kept an accurate assessment of their eating habits. Looking back over their diaries, how would you advise them to change their diets to improve their health? Are there any "red flags" in terms of poor food choices in these food diaries? What choices did Julie and Lilly make that you think are healthy? Do their food choices give you any ideas that you may want to incorporate into your own diet? (I learned from Julie that apples and peanut butter are an awesome combination!) We'll discuss how to evaluate your own food diary in much more detail in Chapter 5, but sometimes I find that it is easier to be more objective in evaluating other people's food choices. So, it may be beneficial to look over these examples provided and think about how these diets could be improved.

To Weigh or Not to Weigh?

At the beginning of this chapter, I advised that you assess your weight and height and take inventory of your weight status. Although it is valuable to assess your weight status before you begin a new eating and exercise regimen and I believe it is worthwhile to step on the scale every month or so, I strongly advise against daily weigh-ins. Weighing your-self daily focuses your attention on a single number. This single number should not be the sole determinant of your success (or lack of) in your weight loss and management efforts.

Research supplies somewhat contradictory evidence about the benefits of weight monitoring (i.e., regular weigh-ins). Patients with eating disor-ders are often advised against monitoring their weight (or strictly forbid-den by a treatment team) because maintaining a healthy weight over time is the goal. The exact number indicating these patients' weight on any given day may be a source of extreme psychological distress. However, a recent study indicated that women and men may respond differently to frequent weight monitoring.[12] In this study, women who weighed them-selves often experienced high levels of preoccupation with their weight and appearance in general. These women expressed greater concern about their body shape than did women who did not weigh themselves more frequently. In contrast, men who weighed themselves frequently indicated greater satisfaction with their bodies and more positive evaluations of their health than men who did not weigh themselves frequently. The way this study was conducted, it is impossible to determine what came first—the frequent weighing or the way men and women felt about their bodies. However, it is possible to speculate that men who were physically fit and felt good about themselves weighed in more often as a means of validating their positive self-image. In contrast, women who were concerned about their weight and already upset about how they looked may have weighed themselves with the hopes of having these concerns refuted with positive feedback from the scale. Regardless of how you interpret the findings from this study, they suggest that frequent weigh-ins may be a source of distress for some people, especially women.

Plus, I maintain that the measure of your success should not be a number on a scale. Focusing on a number distracts you from what you should really be focusing on: How do you feel now? How do you want to feel? Perhaps you want your clothes to feel looser. Maybe you want to have more energy. Generally, you likely want to feel healthier. These outcomes are better metrics of success than is a single number on a scale.

Once you settle into a healthier pattern of eating and exercising and you feel more secure about a long-term approach to weight management, I'll invite you to weigh yourself once a month. Research suggests this may be helpful in long-term weight management, but for right now stay off the scale.[13] I'm happy to admit that there is not a scale to be found anywhere in my house, and I'm glad not to be tempted to check what I weigh regularly. I know when my clothes feel tighter or my belly feels bloated. If I am curious or concerned about what I weigh, then I step on the scale at a health club, doctor's office, or even a friend's bathroom.

Hopefully, about now, you are surprised at how easy this approach to weight loss and weight management seems. Phase 1 is all about taking inventory and getting to know yourself—a critical first step. There should be no sense of deprivation when you follow the instructions for Phase 1. Phase 2 is when you'll start to actually make changes to your eating behaviors. But you'll be happy to hear that there should be no sense of deprivation when you follow the instructions for Phase 2, either! But, before we move on to Phase 2, the next chapter discusses another element of getting to know yourself before embarking on changes to your life: your body image.

- In this chapter, you learned how to assess your own weight status (BMI).
- You now understand how to think about realistic, achievable goals for weight loss and weight management. One of the most important things you can do when embarking on any change to your eating or physical activity is to set reasonable goals!
- You learned about the importance of honestly keeping a food diary for a week before you proceed with Phase 2 (Chapter 5).

STAY **SMART**

Love Yourself Naked

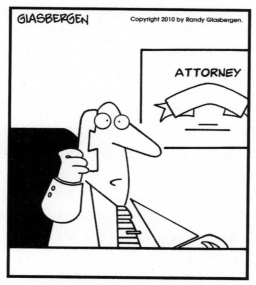

"Well, we can try, Ma'am. But to my knowledge, nobody has ever sued a dressing room mirror before."

Enjoy your body, use it every way you can. Don't be afraid of it, or what other people think of it, it's the greatest instrument you'll ever own.

Kurt Vonnegut

Think about the last time you looked, or peeked, at yourself naked in the mirror. (Don't pretend you've never done this.) Maybe you were deliberately checking yourself out, or maybe you just caught a glimpse of yourself as you got out of the shower. Perhaps, in this moment of stark exposure, you wondered, "Whose butt is that?" Followed by, "Ugh, why can't it be just a little bit smaller?" Or maybe you wished that your biceps were a little less flimsy and a little more defined and that your belly was more flat than round. Have you ever wondered where this voice comes from and why you desire these physical qualities? Maybe a romantic partner once said to you, "Gee, I wish your butt/arms/tummy was smaller." (If so, I hope this is an ex–romantic partner!) But, more likely, no one has ever explicitly told you how you are supposed to look to be deemed attractive. That is, no one except *you*.

So, what is body image? "Body image" is the term that is used to describe our thoughts and feelings about our bodies. If you are happy with your body, then you have what researchers refer to as "body satisfaction." It is a rare person who is truly satisfied with his or her body. Instead, most of us experience some level of *body dissatisfaction*. We wish we were thinner, taller, more muscular, less muscular, had longer legs— you get the idea. Among girls and women, body dissatisfaction is so common that it has long been referred to as a "normative discontent."[1] In other words, body dissatisfaction among girls and women is described as "the new normal." This isn't to say that it is okay that so many of us are not happy with our bodies, just that it is, sadly, the norm. Increasingly, boys and men are also experiencing body dissatisfaction. In my research, I've found that up to 90 percent of girls and women report experiencing body dissatisfaction and up to 75 percent of boys and men report experiencing body dissatisfaction.[2]

Sometimes, body image is measured using simple pictorial measures like the ones below.

Give it a try. Look at the pictures and select the one that you think looks most like you. Now, select the one that you'd most like to look

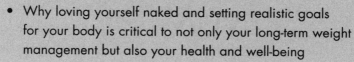

In this chapter you will learn . . .

- How body image is an important component of weight loss and weight management
- How the "myth of transformation" leads us to maintain unrealistic standards for our own bodies
- Why loving yourself naked and setting realistic goals for your body is critical to not only your long-term weight management but also your health and well-being

BECOME
SMART

like. The extent to which there is a discrepancy between these two ratings is used as a rough (but usually very reliable) indication of body dissatisfaction. In my research, it is typical for the average person to indicate that they wished they were one to two pictures smaller than they actually are.[3] I wouldn't be surprised or particularly alarmed if you

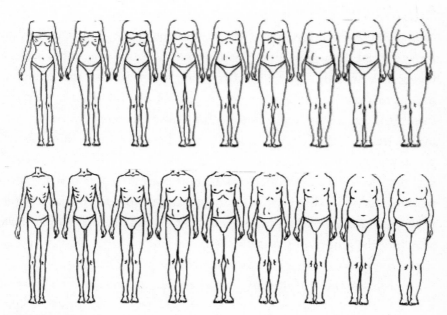

Body Image Pictorial Measure (Thompson & Gray, 1995)[4]

would like to be a picture or two smaller. This is quite normal. However, if you find yourself identifying the picture at the far right as what you look like and the picture at the far left as what you'd want to look like, then your body dissatisfaction is pretty high, and I hope that you pay close attention to the advice I offer in this chapter (if for no other reason than the pictures on the far left are indicative of underweight figures that are not necessarily healthy). By the way, the pictures are headless for a reason; the idea is to get people to focus on the bodies and not be distracted by the faces.

A waist is a terrible thing to mind.

—**Tom Wilson, cartoonist**

Manage Your Image

One of the keys to long-term weight loss and management is to first achieve a certain degree of body satisfaction, a certain amount of acceptance of your body. We all need to come to terms with the fact that weight loss does not change some aspects of our bodies. If you have short legs, you will still have short legs, no matter how much weight you lose. I realize that this may sound somewhat backward. Most likely, you're reading this book because you are not satisfied with how you look and feel. So it may not initially make much sense to hear that I advise working on improving your body image, and to some degree accepting what you currently weigh, prior to starting a weight-loss plan or at least as part of the process of managing your weight long-term. But, trust me, there's a method to what sounds like madness.

It probably isn't too surprising to learn that individuals who are dissatisfied with their bodies tend to be concerned about their own weight and these concerns often lead to dieting behaviors.[5] I know what you are thinking—no duh! No one has "accidently" found themselves on a diet if they were not first concerned about their weight. However, this is where things get a little more complex. Individuals who have high levels of *weight concerns* tend to approach weight management in a maladaptive way, resorting to drastic approaches to weight loss that are not healthy and not likely to be sustainable over the long term.[6] They are prone to skipping meals, eliminating food groups from their diet, binging, and even sometimes purging. In the short run, these strategies might pay off in the sense that a person may lose some weight. The problem (you knew there was going to be one, right?) is that eventually people get hungry (it is tough to skip breakfast every day) or they miss the food they vowed to give up (think chips, cookies, and ice cream) and they find themselves with a cookie (or ten) in their mouth. Weight gain often follows and so do additional concerns about their weight.

Decades of research shows a reciprocal relationship between body image and weight.[7] The reality is that individuals with lower levels of body satisfaction are less successful at losing weight than those with higher levels of body satisfaction. Similar research has found that improvements in body image lead to healthier eating and exercise behaviors. Quite simply, when people feel good about themselves, they are more apt to take good care of themselves, eat well, and exercise.

Getting in the right frame of mind for weight loss and management—and not being down on yourself—is an important part of my advice, whether you want to lose five pounds or twenty-five. To understand the extent to which you are psychologically ready for successful and sustainable weight loss, try completing the exercise below. Be honest with yourself (no one else has to see your answers), and be prepared to work on both your body and mind as you work on weight loss and management. Of course, if you find that you are not in the best state of mind about your weight, there is no reason both your mind and your body can't become more "fit" as you proceed with my advice in the chapters ahead.

Assess Your Weight Concerns

The Weight Concerns Scale is a survey that has been used for nearly two decades in psychological research aimed at understanding individuals' feelings about their weight.[8] Try taking the survey, add up your score, and then look below for information about how to interpret it.

1) How much more or less do you feel you worry about your weight and body shape than other people your age?

   0. I worry a lot less than other people.

   1. I worry a little less than other people.

   2. I worry about the same as other people.

   3. I worry a little more than other people.

   4. I worry a lot more than other people.

2) How afraid are you of gaining three pounds?

   0. I'm not afraid of gaining three pounds.

   1. I'm slightly afraid of gaining three pounds.

   2. I'm moderately afraid of gaining three pounds.

   3. I'm very afraid of gaining three pounds.

   4. I'm terrified of gaining three pounds.

3) Have you ever gone on a diet?

   0. No.

   1. I have gone on a diet once before.

   2. I have gone on more than one diet before.

4) Compared to other things in your life, how important is your weight to you?

   0. My weight is not important compared to other things in my life.

   1. My weight is a little less important than some other things in my life.

   2. My weight is as important as other things in my life.

   3. My weight is more important than most, but not all, things in my life.

   4. My weight is the most important thing in my life.

5) Do you ever feel fat?

   0. Never

   1. Rarely

   2. Sometimes

   3. Often

   4. Always

Scoring: As you may have been able to guess, higher scores are indicative of higher levels of weight concerns. In my research examining adult women in their twenties and thirties, we typically find an average score around 8.[9] There is not an empirically supported cutoff score indicating that an individual has weight concerns that are truly problematic. However, in my professional opinion, a healthy weight concerns score is less than 6. Yes, that is less than the average, meaning that most people (or at least most women) may manifest an unhealthy degree of weight concerns.

> *Our body is . . . a vehicle for awakening. Treat it with care.*
> **—Buddha**

Get Real

How did you score on the Weight Concerns Scale? Even if your score is above average (i.e., you have more weight concerns than you'd like to), it is possible to turn your dissatisfaction into satisfaction and accept your imperfect body. I'm not going to pretend this is easy; we live in a culture obsessed with physical perfection. I don't wake up each day loving my body either. I've never really liked my legs; most days, I accept them, but I can't say I'd mind if they were longer, thinner, and looked a lot more like Gwyneth Paltrow's! From magazines to movies, we are all exposed to an extraordinary number of images of "perfect" bodies. If you are at all in touch with popular culture, you have seen celebrities like Ryan Gosling, Brad Pitt, Angelina Jolie, and Jessica Alba nearly naked. Inevitably, seeing people like this makes us feel bad (at least a little bit) about our bodies.[10] To obtain a body like any of those celebrities is extremely unlikely for any of us. You cannot diet your way into a celebrity body. Even with expensive cosmetic surgery, a personal trainer, a personal chef, and the best approach to weight management around (this one, of course!), most of us will never have the "perfect" body. In fact, most celebrities do not have perfect bodies either. The way we see them—in dramatically made-up, touched-up, and photoshopped form—is not an accurate representation of how *they* really look! Most of us simply do not have on-screen, Hollywood bodies—even the Hollywood celebs themselves. The sooner we get comfortable with this fact and accept realistic goals for weight loss, the happier we will be.

Truly, a certain degree of acceptance goes a long way. Most women will never have Jennifer Lopez's derriere, and most men will never have

David Beckham's six-pack. Of course, if you want to live in the gym and you want to watch every particle of food that passes your lips, you may get close. However, this is not a realistic lifestyle for most of us. And thank goodness—that's a lot of work and pressure! Most of us are students, parents, professionals, and citizens involved in our communities. In short, we have roles and responsibilities that prohibit us (or at least probably should prohibit us) from spending the majority of our time focused on our bodies and weight. Life is way too short, and busy, to obsess about our bodies.

Ignore Media "Thinspiration"

It is hard to resist the draw of those *People* magazine covers as you wait in line at the grocery store. Some celebrity has always just recently lost her baby weight or worked on achieving big biceps for his new movie role. I often find myself thinking, "Why do I care how much Kim Kardashian currently weighs?" However, I sometimes find myself reading in line about her boyfriend or husband (what is it this week?) and her recent weight gain or weight loss. Although not particularly intellectually stimulating, I like to think that these magazine headlines, images, and stories are harmless fun.

However, psychological research provides convincing evidence that this assumption is wrong.[11] Exposure to "idealized media images" (e.g., the pictures on those magazine covers) leads to decreases in body satisfaction among adolescents and adults.[12] Perhaps even more disturbing is research indicating that celebrities are particularly influential on teenagers' feelings about their bodies.[13] This contributes to body dissatisfaction, decreases in self-esteem, increases in depression, and vulnerability to eating disorders.[14]

It's not only these magazines but also the television shows we watch that influence our body image. In research done in my lab, shows that feature physical makeovers have been found to be detrimental to viewers' feelings about their own physical appearance.[15] For example, people who watched *Extreme Makeover*, in which a woman's physical appearance is radically transformed (e.g., through cosmetic surgery), were more likely to desire having plastic surgery themselves! Not only did these individuals want to alter their own bodies but they also believed that doing so would make them look significantly better and would make them happier—just like the woman on the show. These sorts of results have been replicated and strongly suggest that individuals who routinely engage with the media are being trained to view changing their appearance as the key to success and happiness.

So, should we stop reading *People* and watching TV? This is probably not a realistic solution to improving body image for most of us. Some researchers suggest that parents may be wise to restrict their children's access to some media and that parents should use media (e.g., television coviewing) with their children to improve their children's healthy attitudes and behaviors about their bodies.[16] For the rest of us bombarded with several thousand ads per day, we need to consciously remind ourselves that these images can be detrimental to our well-being.[17] And, anyway, the myth that changing yourself physically in some way will change your entire life is just that—a myth. It's a fairytale that we were taught at a very young age.

My Beef with Barbie

Even though I consider myself a feminist, I like to do "girly" activities with my daughter. We paint our fingernails together, I do her hair, and we go clothes shopping. However, there is one typical "girl thing" I don't condone: Barbie dolls are not allowed in our home. My daughter hates this rule, and I'm sure at least a few of our friends find it fairly strange (or at least rigid) of me. But before you throw your Malibu Ken or pink corvette at me, let me explain myself.

Barbie dolls epitomize the exact figure that girls grow up wanting and boys grow up wanting their girlfriends (and someday wives) to have. However,

Barbie's small waist, large breasts, never mind the arched feet and complete hairlessness, would leave a real woman unable to stand, much less function. Some have estimated that in real life Barbie would be six feet tall and weigh a hundred pounds. However, when scientists carefully evaluate Barbie, with a height of 5'7", her bust-waist-hip measurements would be 32–16–29.[18] Even with breast implants, liposuction, and a good corset, most women are simply not going to be able to achieve these proportions.[19]

Just like magazines and movies, research indicates that Barbie impacts our children's views of thinness and body esteem (body esteem is similar to body image but focuses on how people *feel* about their bodies).[20] In one study, girls ages five to eight were either exposed to images of Barbie, an Emme doll (US size 16; modeled after real-life plus-size model, Emme), or no doll. The girls who were in the Barbie group were more interested in being thin and reported lower body esteem than the girls in the Emme- and no-doll groups.

My daughter is only getting older, and I don't worry that playing with a Barbie doll every now and then will completely warp her views of femininity. But, doing what I do for a living, I have to take a stand. At the end of the day, what is most important to me is dialogue with our children about body image. I tell my daughter, "Real women don't look like Barbies," and, "I don't want you to ever think that you need to look like a Barbie," and, "You are beautiful just the way you are," and, "What's in your brain is more important than what you look like." I hope that someday she looks back, understands the "no Barbie rule," and her own body image benefits. Or, perhaps, she'll just become so infatuated with this toy that she's not allowed to have that she'll end up working for Mattel.

The Myth of Transformation

Most diet plans and countless other beauty aids target your insecurities and aim to make you feel bad about yourself. Your arms are too flabby, your penis is too small, your gut is too big, or your butt is too round.

The marketing message behind a whole host of products—bras, penis enlargement products, and, of course, diet aids—is fairly simple: you are imperfect and should be unhappy, but this product will make you closer to perfect and will make you happier. You are being sold what body-image researchers refer to as the "myth of transformation." If you attempt to transform yourself physically—typically via expensive and often ineffective products—not only will you look better, but everything about your life will be better. The illusion is very tempting and these products proliferate. We all want to improve ourselves and we all want to be happy. The trick is setting realistic goals when it comes to physical improvement and understanding what products are merely playing on our insecurities about our physical selves.

Have you ever gotten a new haircut and thought that you looked pretty darn good? Maybe you got compliments the first week. Maybe you felt better about your appearance in general after you got this haircut. However, chances are the self-esteem boost following this haircut was short lived. I'm guessing that this new haircut did not help you land a promotion or new job. It probably didn't help you get a new boyfriend or girlfriend. It probably didn't really make you a happier person for more than a few hours or maybe (if it was a really great haircut) a couple of days. Researchers who study individuals after they undergo cosmetic surgery actually find a similar pattern. People who get a nose job tend to like their nose better following their procedure and may feel better about themselves in general for a few months.[21] However, over time, there is little evidence to suggest that "fixing" your nose will fix your entire life. Thinking any different is succumbing to the myth of transformation, the myth that changing yourself physically in some way will change your entire life. If only life were that simple. Even celebrities we admire have imperfections. Accepting our imperfections will not only keep us from weight obsession but will make us happier. This is important, given that research suggests that looking "perfect" is unlikely to lead to long-term happiness anyway.

Even the models we see in magazines wish they could look like their own images.

—Cheri K. Erdman, author of Live Large

Fake Out

The influence of the media on our body image and related weight concerns is especially worrisome given the dishonest messages presented in the media. The majority of the media images we view have been altered. In fact, among people "in the industry" it is widely accepted that photographs will be edited, retouched, and, in many cases, dramatically altered. A head can be put on a different body. A body can be stretched to slenderize it. Breasts can be made larger; cellulite and wrinkles can be "erased." Photo manipulation has developed into an art form in and of itself. However, it has recently been acknowledged that these photos are misleading and potentially harmful to the viewer, prompting some discussion about labeling photos that have been manipulated.

In a recent study, fashion magazine photos were presented to groups of young women.[22] Some women saw the photographs as they would in a magazine, whereas other women saw the same photographs but with "warning" labels indicating the pictures had been digitally altered. Women who viewed photos with warning labels reported more body satisfaction than did the women who viewed photos without labels. Findings such as these have led the American Medical Association to take a stand against excessive photo retouching as a threat to public health.[23] Some celebrities, such as Jamie Lee Curtis, Kate Winslet, and Nigella Lawson have even asked that photographs of them *not* be retouched, in an effort to combat the detrimental effects of "false advertising" in photography.

The excessive use of retouching of photography has prompted the National Press Photographers Association to develop a code of ethics demanding integrity and accuracy in photographs used in advertising. Specifically, this code insists that photographers "do not manipulate images . . . that can mislead viewers or misrepresent subjects."[24] Unfortunately, all photographers and advertisers have not taken this call for accuracy to heart. In 2009, an ad for Ralph Lauren featuring the beautiful model Fillipa Hamilton caused an uproar because the image of her was altered so much that her head appeared to be larger than her pelvis.[25] The same year, an ad featuring the iconic model Twiggy prompted discussion in the United Kingdom about banning retouching in photos. Twiggy was retouched for an antiaging skin-care product to suggest that she had hardly any wrinkles—even at fifty-nine years of age. Ultimately, the Advertising Standards Authority banned this particular magazine advertisement, but this single case of action against false advertising does little to put a dent in the myriad fake images we all view daily.[26]

An Interview with Eric Bauer, Photographer, http://visionsofnature.wix.com/elbweddingphotography

Eric Bauer is a professional photographer with more than fifteen years of experience photographing architecture, products, portraits, sports, corporate events, and weddings. He received a master's degree in photography from the prestigious Brooks Institute of Photography in Santa Barbara, California. Below are some excerpts from an interview that I conducted with him.

CM: When you take pictures for media publications do you retouch the pictures?

EB: Nearly 100 percent of the time pictures used in media publications are retouched by a professional retoucher. Usually, a photographer will take the pictures and then pass them on to another professional. What most people don't realize is that there are people who make a living just editing and retouching photos.

CM: In your professional opinion, what percentage of pictures displayed in popular publications (e.g., *People* magazine) have been retouched?

EB: 99.99 percent of the time these photos are retouched; unless perhaps the goal is to make people look unattractive.

CM: Do you think that media pictures and advertisements are deceptive, and, if so, is there a moral problem with this? Do you think that photographers should have to provide labels or "fine print" indicating when photographs have been altered?

EB: Photographs are altered and often deceptive when the goal is selling a product, and this is morally wrong. Young people in particular don't realize that the images that they see are fake, and this may affect their views of themselves. If the health and well-being of younger people in society could be protected by disclaimers, then this could be a good idea. However, I don't expect that the industry will necessarily cooperate with the inclusion of photo labels, particularly in the fashion industry. It is different when photos are altered to create fine art. It is the photographer's prerogative to take what exists in real life and make it more beautiful.

How to Get a Handle on Body Angst

Because the media surrounds us with so many negative messages about our bodies, it can feel like a losing battle—how can we possibly love ourselves naked when we are so imperfect? Instead of looking in the mirror and pointing out your flaws, spend time focusing on the parts of your physical self that you *do* like. Maybe you have good hair, nice lips, muscular calves, big eyes, or handsome feet. Whenever you are tempted to be self-critical, think about the physical features that you feel good about, and remind yourself that complete perfection is impossible but self-acceptance is not.

Let me ask you something, in all the years that you have . . . undressed in front of a gentleman has he ever asked you to leave? Has he ever walked out and left? No? It's because he doesn't care! He's in a room with a naked girl, he just won the lottery.

—Elizabeth Gilbert, author

In addition to spending time focusing on the positive, here are some commonsense (and in most cases, scientifically proven) ways to ease your body angst:

- **Exercise.** Plenty of research suggests that physical activity leads to improvements in body image.[27] I know from personal experiences that when I exercise regularly I not only feel fit and strong; I also feel better about my body in general. Not only may exercise improve your physical fitness, but it can help you to value your body for something other than how it looks—how it moves.
- **Avoid the mirror.** Although it is probably advisable to spend some amount of time using a mirror for basic grooming practices (hair brushing, makeup application, etc.), there is no need to spend a lot of time in front of the mirror each day. Spending time checking yourself out inevitably leads to scrutiny ("Why aren't my legs thinner, my butt smaller, my abs more defined?"), and scrutiny leads to a depressed mood.[28] So give yourself a quick glance before you leave the house to be sure you don't have food in your teeth or hair standing on end, and move on to more important things.
- **Focus on other attributes.** It's important to remind yourself that you have many positive qualities besides your physical attributes.

Focus your attention on these other attributes. If you're having a hard time identifying them, ask a friend. I have a friend who is always stylish and well put together, yet she is constantly worried about her weight. I try to remind her that not only does she look great but she has so many other qualities that I value her for: she's funny, kind, a wonderful friend, and an excellent shopping companion. This is good advice, as research has found that focusing on our physical appearance distracts us from matters that we may value more. For example, in one study, researchers tried to force young women to think about their physical appearance by having them try on and wear bathing suits while other participants tried on a sweaters. To test the "comfort" of these clothing items, the women were asked to take a math test while they wore them. The women wearing a bathing suit did worse on the math test than those who were wearing the sweaters. Why? Feeling physically vulnerable and thinking about our physical selves seems to be very distracting. Just imagine what we all could accomplish if we spent less time thinking about how we look.[29]

- **Keep good company.** The company we keep plays an important role in our body image and related concerns. Women who have weight concerns influence their friends to also have weight concerns. In contrast, women who talk about exercise with their friends have more positive body images.[30] The bottom line seems to be that it makes sense to spend time with other people who are health conscious but not obsessed with their bodies or frequently engaged in fad diets. I'm not necessarily suggesting that you dump your friends who have a poor body image, but it does make sense to be aware of the effect they could have on you. No one can ever have too many friends, and making an effort to have friends with healthier attitudes about their bodies is advisable.

Are Self-Acceptance and Health at Odds with Each Other?

The message in this book is that we need to lose weight to be healthy but we should also accept some of our physical imperfections. These are not necessarily contradictory messages. When you appreciate yourself—even your imperfections—you will be much more capable of improving yourself and sticking to the regimen for weight loss that I prescribe.

A certain degree of self-acceptance—even self-forgiveness—is conducive to both mental and physical health. Sometimes, I tell my students to "talk to themselves in a gentler way" and treat their bodies like they would treat a good friend. Would you tell your friend he or she is fat? If you spend a lot of energy upset with yourself, frustrated with your weight, and distraught about your appearance, a logical response will be to do something drastic to improve yourself. However, healthy weight management is not drastic; it is gradual. To embark on a long-term approach to weight management, you need to be patient with yourself. It doesn't hurt to acknowledge that your weight is just one aspect of your life and that you should appreciate yourself for your many other qualities and capabilities.

I cannot pretend that patience and self-acceptance is always easy to come by. There are countless daily messages that tell us we need to improve some part of our physical selves. There are countless products, procedures, and diet plans available that claim to give us physical perfection. These quick fix tricks are appealing because they promise us improvements that we so desperately want. But, if we accept ourselves a bit, we won't need these tricks.

Value Your Body, Value Your Health

Feeling good about our bodies is important to both our mental and physical health.[31] But feeling good about our bodies means adopting a realistic view of our bodies. We must be kinder to ourselves than we typically are. We must stop looking for our flaws and start to remind ourselves of our features that we *do* like. Try to embrace the elements of your physical self that make you a unique human being. People simply come in all different shapes and sizes.

This is a call to arms. A call to be gentle, to be forgiving, to be generous with yourself. The next time you look into the mirror, try to let go of the story line that says you're too fat or too shallow, too ashy or too old, your eyes are too small or your nose too big; just look into the mirror and see your face. When the criticism drops away, what you will see then is just you, without judgment, and that is the first step toward transforming your experience of the world.

—Oprah Winfrey

It also helps to view our bodies as more than something that we "display" physically. Our bodies have a functional purpose and not just an aesthetic purpose. We tend to take our functionality for granted until we injure ourselves or aging prohibits activities that used to be possible. If you've ever broken a foot and found yourself unable to walk or if you have back problems and find yourself uncomfortable often, then you know what I mean when I say that the function of our bodies is far more important than the way they look. Some days, I have to remind myself that, in spite of my many physical imperfections, I can run farther now than I ever have been able to in my life. With middle age around the corner, I find a lot of comfort in knowing that my body is strong and fit; I'm pretty sure I could beat Gwyneth Paltrow in just about any race!

We may live in a looks-obsessed culture, but we don't need to let vanity obscure common sense. Commonsense values health and fitness above looks. I want to help you love yourself naked by arming you with the tools to lose weight sustainably and generally improve your overall health and functionality. I want you to look better, feel better, and move better than you ever have, and for many years to come.

- Feeling good about our bodies may result from weight loss, but feeling good about our bodies will also make weight loss more possible—it is all about setting appropriate expectations and goals.
- The bodies we compare our own to are often fake; we have to adopt realistic expectations for our own bodies.
- This book is not about getting you the "perfect" body, because such a thing does not exist. It is about getting you a healthy, fit body that you can love naked.

STAY SMART

Bite by Bite

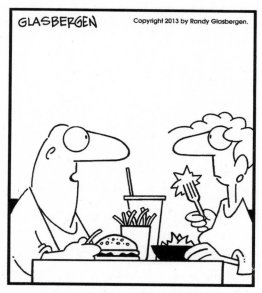

"**Sticking to my diet is hard work.
I can't do it on an empty stomach!**"

Success is the sum of small efforts, repeated day in and day out.

Robert Collier, author

You have now weighed in and have a realistic view of how you measure up. You've also begun the daily work of accepting yourself for who you are and what you weigh today. Now, it's time to take a closer look at your food and exercise routines and how you can begin to shift them toward healthier habits that you're willing to adopt for a lifetime. For starters, what do you think of your eating habits? What are you happy about and what would you like to change? Look back over what you recorded after reading Chapter 3, "Honestly Weigh In," and identify your healthy food choices (fruit, vegetables) versus your unhealthy food choices (French fries, candy) and the extent to which you are physically active. Now, get ready to make some changes!

Every Bite Counts (Over Time)

The goal is not to eliminate all your unhealthy food choices; a life without cake may not be worth living. The goal is to identify healthy food that you can see yourself regularly eating and enjoying and to identify physical activities that you will regularly do more of or be willing to add to your daily routine. You need to establish healthy habits that can be sustained across the rest of your life. By the way, healthy habits can include some cake and even some cookies, ice cream, and candy—in moderation. It is not necessary to eat "perfectly" to be healthy, and you're likely to be happier and more dedicated to a healthy lifestyle if you keep your expectations reasonable.

An evidence-based approach to change unhealthy habits and create healthy habits is to do so very gradually. To actually achieve your goals, you need to start by setting small, obtainable goals.[1] Goals such as cutting out snacks or sweets entirely are nearly impossible for most people to achieve and are unlikely to be sustainable. So, you need to begin by making one minor change to your diet per week until you are satisfied with your new eating regimen. For some people, this may mean making one minor change every week for ten weeks. Others may feel like they

In this chapter you will learn . . .

- How to systematically think about and improve your typical eating and physical activity habits
- How to change *one habit one week at a time* to gradually lose weight and improve your health
- The importance of patience, diligence, and long-term thinking as you embark on Phase 2. Depending on how much weight you want to lose or how many habits you want to change, this phase may take you three weeks or three months—it's up to you!

BECOME
SMART

are on the right track after just three or four weeks. You'll know that you are "done" establishing new habits when you've reached a (realistic) goal weight and when you feel healthier and happier. This approach will not lead to immediate, dramatic weight loss, but immediate, dramatic weight loss is not sustainable weigh loss. Remember, quick-fix diets don't work and often result in weight gain, not loss. Don't let yourself fall for the frustration involved in fad dieting. You are trying to change your habits to *promote weight loss and improved health for the rest of your life.*

On the following pages you will find suggestions for altering your eating habits. As you read over these suggestions, look back at the food diary you completed following my advice in Chapter 3. Think about your current food habits and what you could realistically eliminate from your daily routine. Remember, you do not have to give up any foods forever, just remove some unhealthy options from your *daily* eating habits. I'll explain how you can replace unhealthy choices with a healthy alternative for one week. At the end of the week, you should ask yourself whether you can honestly live with this change. If so, then move on to the next item. Remember, this isn't a race. Take your time and focus on just one food item alteration per week.

I do want to provide one word of caution: throughout this chapter I will discuss calories (and a more in-depth discussion of calories can be found in Chapter 7). Although I don't recommend counting calories every day, it is valuable to look at nutritional information when you first establish good nutritional habits. Sometimes, foods that seem healthy are hiding a lot of calories, fat, sugar, or salt and aren't actually healthy at all! Once you know what you both like and is good for you (and in what portion size!), then you won't need to worry about the exact nutritional information in the future. I promise, once you have eliminated unhealthy foods from your diet and settled into good food routines you don't have to focus on the details every day!

DANIELLE'S *Story*

When I started to follow Dr. Markey's advice for weight loss, I think the biggest change I made to my eating habits was breakfast. I used to eat whatever I could get my hands on as I rushed out the door—a muffin, a doughnut, some toast. I did whatever was easiest. Now I plan for my breakfasts when I do my groceries. I make sure that I have easy but healthy options in the house. Some days I have a hard-boiled egg and an English muffin. Some days I make oatmeal and have a banana. I have more energy, and I like starting the day off with a good meal.

Changing what I drank and snacked on was also key to my weight loss. I used to always go for chips in the afternoon, and I actually eat a couple of pieces of fruit instead. I don't run to the vending machine around three o'clock for chips and a soda but am sure to have at least a banana on hand. I also completely cut out regular soda. Some days, I still drink Coke zero, but I try to stick to water as much as possible.

Making one change at a time made all of this easier than any past diet I had tried. I think that getting in the routine of eating a lot of the same foods that I liked, I knew were healthy, were relatively low in calories, and were easy to prepare was a big part of this for me. I was amazed when the weight gradually kept coming off! Twenty pounds in a little over two months and over a year later I still haven't gained it back!

~**Danielle,** AGE THIRTY-THREE, NURSE

The Less-Liquid Diet

The easiest, most efficient way to drop calories and other undesirable nutrients (e.g., sugar) from your diet is to change what you drink. If you already drink water 80 percent of the time and low-fat (or nonfat) milk the other 20 percent of the time, then you can skip this section. But because most of us do not consume liquids in these proportions, I encourage you to stay put and read on.

Many of us don't count beverages as a part of our diet; if it is not a solid, it is often overlooked and "guilt free." However, the greatest culprit in adding nonnutritive calories to American's diets is drinkable, in particular, soda and other sugar-sweetened beverages (e.g., juice, sports drinks, and energy drinks).[2] I'll concede that most of these beverages taste good, and if you're in the habit of consuming them, it may seem hard to stop. However, "drinking your calories" is one of the least satisfying ways to consume calories, and yet it's one of the fastest ways to put weight on. Soda and sugar-sweetened beverages are estimated to contribute more to the rise in obesity than are any other single food or beverage item.[3] This is one of the reasons some cities and states have discussed taxing soda and even banning large portions of these drinks. A twelve-ounce soda contains approximately 150 calories and thirty-nine grams of sugar. Of course, most sodas are not sold or consumed in twelve-ounce containers, so if you purchase a Big Gulp, you'll be getting thirty-two ounces, close to 400 calories, and more than *ninety* grams of sugar. Most reasonable breakfasts contain around 400 calories (often less for women), so would you rather have breakfast or a big soda with lunch? Hopefully, that's an easy choice for you (hint: go with breakfast!).

Unfortunately, juice is not much better for us than is soda (it falls into the sugar-sweetened beverages category, in spite of manufacturers' claims to be "real" in many cases). For example, one of my personal favorites, cranberry-grape juice, contains 140 calories per cup (that's only eight ounces) and thirty-five grams of sugar. Unlike soda, there is a bit of nutritional value in many juices, but the labeling of many juices is extremely deceptive; you're likely getting much less fruit than the advertising would lead you to believe. Cranberry juice is popularly known as having health benefits for the bladder, a claim that is only somewhat true. Ingredients present in pure, unsweetened cranberry juice help prevent bacterial adherence to the bladder walls, reducing the likelihood of infection. In effect, the acidity of cranberries causes the bladder to empty regularly (a sensitive or damaged bladder will actually be worsened by consumption of cranberry juice). But most commercial cranberry juices have added sugar and next to no health benefits. Orange juice contains high doses of vitamins C and B and is often fortified with calcium, but eight ounces still contain about 110 calories and twenty-two grams of sugar. You'd be much better off having a glass of water and eating a real orange (60 calories, twelve grams of sugar, and fiber to boot!).

Alcoholic drinks and coffee beverages are another source of unnecessary calories. Many of us don't consider that a standard glass of wine contains about five ounces and 120 calories. That twelve-ounce beer might taste good, but it is also around 150 calories. A martini, depending on the exact ingredients used to make it, may range from about 120 to 300 calories for about five ounces. Similarly, and most sad to this margarita lover, is the caloric content of margaritas, ranging from about 150 calories to 300, depending on the exact ingredients and portion size. How about your daily dose of Starbucks? A regular cup of coffee, without cream or sugar, may have as few as 5 calories. But, a white chocolate mocha (sixteen ounces) contains about 400.

The Skinny on Soda

Perhaps no other (legal) ingestible substance has received as much research attention, speculation, and policy consideration in recent years as soda. This focus on soda appears to be warranted. It has been estimated that approximately half the US population over the age of two consumes soda on a daily basis.[4] In fact, there is a good chance that almost 10 percent of your caloric intake can be attributed to it.[5] Soda consumption has been linked to the rise in obesity rates in the United States and appears to be associated with the recent increase in type 2 diabetes.[6]

Hundreds of studies have examined links between soda consumption and weight status. One study of 500,000 adolescents in California found a strong link between obesity rates and the proximity of kids' schools to fast-food establishments.[7] How is soda relevant? Adolescents who had easy access to McDonald's, Taco Bell, or a similar restaurant were less likely to eat fruit and vegetables and *more likely to drink soda*. It wasn't really the fast food that was making them fat; it was the soda! Even those of us who consume diet soda are not immune to the negative effects of these beverages. A recent ten-year study found a convincing link between the consumption of *diet* soda and stroke, myocardial infarction, and vascular death (i.e., cardiovascular disease and related consequences).[8] So, what's a soda lover to do? These studies are not strong endorsements for soda consumption—diet or regular—but they do hint at the complexities uncovered in research examining soda.

Looking at a wide range of studies, it is clear that soda consumption is associated with a number of negative consequences, and this seems to be truer of regular soda than diet soda. *Smart People Don't Diet* is all about using scientific information such as this, making sense of it, and applying it to your own life. Sometimes science meshes well with common sense; you probably already knew that regular soda does not contain any nutritionally beneficial ingredients and is high in sugar and calories. Sometimes, science reveals surprising findings, such as the potential link between *diet* soda and health problems. Regardless, soda isn't the best beverage option available. This bad news still doesn't mean that you can *never* have soda! I think nothing tastes better at a movie theater than popcorn and a Coke, and I have no intention of completely abstaining from my overpriced movie snacks.

Drink Fewer Calories

So, how should you handle all of these drinkable calories with little nutritional value? Well, for your first week of dietary change, try to make
one simple change in your beverage consumption. If you usually have a
white chocolate mocha each day, switch it for a regular cup of coffee or
even a "skinny" or sugar-free flavored latte (180 calories for sixteen
ounces instead of 400). The idea is not to deprive yourself of drinks that
you enjoy but to make healthier choices more regularly. Buy 100 percent
real juice (not the 10 percent fruit juice options that are often 90 percent
sugar!), or if you can, stop buying juice altogether. Switch to seltzer water (0 calories) or mix your juice with seltzer, and you can cut your calorie consumption in half. Instead of regular soda, switch to diet soda. If
the taste is too unpalatable, have a half diet / half regular soda combination. Gradually, try to give up both diet and regular soda altogether
(really, there is nothing healthy about soda). Cut out that glass of wine
in the evenings, and save it for the weekends or special occasions.

Always be careful when you are altering your consumption habits.
You don't want to stop one bad habit and encourage the beginning of a
new bad habit. For example if you completely stop drinking wine during
the weekdays only to start drinking five glasses on Saturdays, this de-
feats the purpose! Start by cutting back in one sustainable way, and as
you do, notice how you feel.

My goal for you is to reduce your caloric intake of nonnutritive beverages by about 200 calories a day—or more if you drink a lot of beverages other than water or milk (low fat and nonfat milk, as well as
nonsweetened, nondairy milks, get a pass because you get a lot of bang
for your buck—they are relatively high in nutritional value and relatively
low in calories). Keep in mind that this is a long-term change you are
aiming for, so make changes you can stick to. Within reason. Dietary
changes don't need to leave you completely inflexible. If you find out on
a Wednesday that you have been promoted at work, go out and have a

nice dinner and a glass of wine to celebrate. However, you shouldn't find a reason to celebrate every Wednesday. If your day feels miserable without the reward of a glass of wine at night, then cutting out that glass of wine may not be a sustainable change for you. Maybe you can cut out the second glass of wine or you can eliminate another beverage you regularly consume. If, after evaluating the drinks you consume, you believe that you don't have changes to make in your beverage consumption, then you have less work to do. However, for most people, starting by altering one drink you consume daily is a relatively easy and effective way to start changing eating behaviors for the better. If you have a lot of room for improvement here (too many fancy coffee drinks, glasses of wine, or juice), then try to make more than one change to your beverage consumption—one week at a time.

Rich was a student who signed up to be in one of my studies, and I worked with him to make dietary changes across a few weeks. He started by eliminating his typical one to two beers with dinner most weekdays. He still had a couple of drinks on the weekend, but he was able to eliminate about 1,000 calories per week by cutting out alcohol and switching to water and diet soda. Similarly, a woman I know, Jane, stopped buying juice and bottled iced tea beverages. She was also able to eliminate about 1,000 calories from her weekly intake by dropping out one of these drinks per day. She switched to seltzer and doesn't miss the old drinks and has ended up being a few dress sizes smaller.

Although what we eat and weigh does involve complex nutritional science, basic math can show how just eliminating a single soda a day can save you calories and help you avoid pounds. The figure below shows how many pounds you'd avoid if you drop a can of soda a day for different periods of time. As you can see, simply eliminating a can of soda for a single day does almost nothing—at most you'd lose .04 pounds (about the weight of three nickels). However, if you kept this up for a month, you could drop 1.25 pounds. Not bad! As you stop desiring this syrupy concoction, *you'll drop about 15 pounds (or 53,000 calories) in*

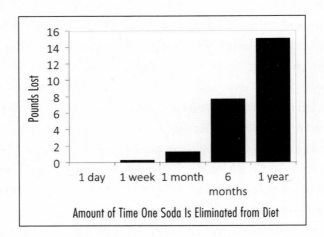

a year! Of course, this assumes that you don't replace soda with another unhealthy beverage or food item. However, it is truly amazing how such a small can of soda can have a dramatic effect on our health across our lifetime.

Cutting calories drink by drink may seem like a really, really slow way to lose weight. Most of us want to cut out all of our unhealthy habits today and lose five pounds *this week*. You want the satisfaction of getting on the scale a week from now and seeing that you weigh noticeably less. Although a dramatic weigh-in may feel like real progress, I encourage you to take it slow and steady. Resist the temptation to move more quickly than I recommend. Remember, you've gone on dramatic diets before, and did they work? This time, try patience. I promise you that patience and persistence is the key to permanently changing your habits, along with your weight. Take a deep breath and read on.

Cut the Snacks

Once you've spent at least one week reducing the amount of calories you're drinking (and maybe a few weeks, depending on how many drink changes you made in your diet), evaluate your snack time. Are you someone who grazes throughout the day—a handful of nuts here, a bag of chips there, a few nibbles of a scone along with a latte before the afternoon meeting? Although many people seem to think that snacks should be eliminated to lose weight, this isn't necessarily true—if your snacks are kept under control! A recent study found that small portions of snacks can be just as satisfying as larger portions.[9] This may not make much sense at first read, but it turns out that our minds have as much to do with how hungry we feel as do our stomachs. In other words, satiety (the feeling of being sated or full) is largely psychological. Consuming a small snack may be all we need to hold us over, so snacking isn't necessarily a bad thing.

The biggest problem with snacking is that most of us eat snacks when we aren't actually hungry. Although we might snack throughout the day, the most popular time for snacking is in the afternoon. During this time of day, our energy levels are lagging, and we look to food to give us a bit of oomph and inspiration. Snacks may provide an important nutritional and psychological mechanism, but the trick is to choose our snacks wisely. The typical vending machine's options can be hard to resist: chips, cookies, candy, and high-sugar energy drinks. As you might guess, these are not wise snacking options. A small bag of potato chips contains about 150 calories (with 60 percent of them derived from fat). A regular bag of peanut M&Ms is 278 calories (with 46 percent derived from fat). Four Oreo cookies are 160 calories (with about 38 percent derived from fat; note that most packs of Oreos contain at least eight cookies or at least 320 calories). Although the caloric content of these sorts of snacks is not terribly large, the fat content is high, and it is unlikely that four Oreos is going to hold you over and make you feel full. In contrast, a banana and an apple (less than 100 calories each and no fat) would be more filling, take you longer to eat, and will be more nutritionally advantageous.

Remember, you should not be concerned about eating a single bag of peanut M&Ms now and then (we all want something sweet sometimes!); my goal for you is to switch out unhealthy snacks that you *regularly* consume for healthier options. The healthiest snack options are fruits and vegetables. Most Americans don't get nearly enough fruit and vegetables in their daily diets.[10] In fact, I often challenge people to try to eat too many fruits and vegetables. (If you happen to be diabetic, don't take me up on this challenge.) It is nearly impossible to do. Most fruits and vegetables are relatively low in caloric content and high in nutritional value. Eat as many as you want as often as you want, and you are very unlikely to gain any weight. If you find yourself craving chips in the afternoon, choose something instead from the list below. There are many options available that are not on this list, but what I've tried to include are options that are relatively nutrient dense and relatively low in calories.

As you can see, most of the best snack options cannot be found in vending machines and often require some amount of preparation. At first, planning snacks to have on hand may seem tedious and tiresome. However, once you get used to always having an apple or a bag of nuts handy, you'll find that you're grateful to avoid having to look for a snack when you get hungry. You will also feel a lot better after eating a healthy apricot, almonds, or even pretzels than you will after downing some Cheetos. To encourage healthy snacking, you should stock up on options that you like and keep them strategically in your car, office, purse, briefcase, or backpack. I always have some of my favorite Luna bars and single-serve microwave popcorn bags in my office. They may not be the *best* snack options, but they offer portion control, they don't perish, they taste good, the calorie count is relatively low, they've gotten me through many afternoons, and they don't leave my fingers covered in orange Cheeto dust (what is that stuff anyway?).

As the following table suggests, altering your snacking means purchasing new items and not purchasing others. If you know that you will snack on chips if they are in the house, don't buy them. If you usually have regular tortilla chips and don't want to give them up, try switching to baked tortilla chips. As with beverages, you want to start by switching one habit at a time. Wait until you feel comfortable with eliminating one bad snacking habit before moving onto the next. If you typically

SUPER SNACKS

Snack ideas	Serving Size	Calories	Fat (g)	Fiber (g)	Protein (g)	Sugar (g)
Almonds	1 oz (28 g)	163	4.6	0.9	2	0.4
Apple	1 medium (182 g)	95	0.3	4.4	0.5	18.9
Applesauce with Pecans	1 cup applesauce (244 g) 1 oz pecans (28 g)	297	78.7	5.4	3	23
Apricot	1 whole (35 g)	79	0.1	0.7	0.5	3.2
Baked Tortilla Chips	10 chips (16 g)	74	2.4	0.9	1.4	0.1
Banana	1 medium (118 g)	105	0.4	3.1	1.3	14.4
Blueberries	1 cup (148 g)	84	0.5	3.6	1.1	14.7
Carrot	1 medium (61 g)	25	0.1	1.7	0.6	2.9
Celery	1 cup, chopped (101 g)	16	0.2	1.6	0.7	1.8
Cottage Cheese	4 oz (113 g)	111	4.9	0	12.6	3
Cracker Chips, Sea Salt	18 chips	80	1.5	2	1	2
Cucumbers	1 cup, sliced (119 g)	14	0.2	0.8	0.7	1.6
Edamame (in pod)	1 cup (155 g)	155	8.1	8.1	16.9	3.4
Fiber Square Cereal	3/4 cup (30 g)	80	1	10	1	3
Granola	1/2 cup (122 g)	140	29.4	11	18.1	24.4
Grapes	1 cup (92 g)	62	0.3	0.8	0.6	14.9
Plain Greek Yogurt	1 packaged cup (245 g)	100	0	0	18	7
Hard-Boiled Egg	1 egg (50 g)	77	5.3	0	6.3	0.6
Hummus	1 tbsp (15 g)	25	1.4	0.9	1.2	0
Instant Oatmeal (Plain)	1/2 cup (40 g)	153	5.3	8.2	10.6	0.8
Orange	1 large (184 g)	86	0.2	4.4	1.7	17.2
Peanut Butter	1 oz (28 g)	146	9.5	1.5	7.3	2.6
Pear	1 large (230 g)	133	0.3	7.1	0.9	22.5
Popcorn	1 single-serving bag, plain (24 g)	93	0.4	1.2	1.0	0.1
Pretzels	1 oz (twenty mini) (28 g)	106	0.7	0.8	2.9	0.8
Raisins	1 miniature box (14 g)	42	0.1	0.5	0.4	8.3
Snow Peas	1 oz (28 g)	12	0.1	0.8	0.9	1.1
Sorbet	1/2 cup, most flavors (97 g)	100	0	0	0	19
Strawberries	1 cup, sliced (152 g)	49	0.5	3	1	7.4
String Cheese	1 piece (28 g)	80	6	0	6	0

Note: All nutritional values provided in this table are based on best estimates, but specifics may vary depending on brands of items or exact size of fruits and vegetables.

find yourself running to the corner store each afternoon, then pack a snack and try to keep yourself away from the store for a week. When in doubt, add in fruit or veggies for snacks. It is likely that you can eat a banana, an apple, *and* some berries in place of a processed snack food and consume fewer calories and benefit more from the higher nutritional value. The trick is to find snacks that you like—and want to eat—that are also good for you. Get in the habit of eating these new snacks most of the time. You want to focus on making changes to your eating behaviors that you can imagine sustaining for the rest of your life, not just until swimsuit season begins.

Nicole was a student in my Psychology of Eating class who was encouraged to switch out an afternoon Snickers bar (in spite of the advertising claim that it "really satisfies") for one Nature Valley granola bar. This amounted to about a 150-calorie reduction in her food intake every day. That's 1050 less calories per week just from switching out one snack, and she was more than satisfied! Another student, Rob, a fruit lover, was happy to eliminate chips from his morning routine by replacing them with an apple *and* an orange. This simple change saved him a few hundred calories every week, while significantly increasing his weekly nutritional intake. You see, if you *reduce 150 calories from your diet each day* (or one bag of chips), that's 4,500 calories over the course of a month. Across the year, that would be 54,000 calories, or a reduction of *more than 15 pounds*. The idea is to make these relatively minor modifications to your regular diet without constantly feeling like you need to track what you eat. In other words, don't count calories, fat, or carbs once you start to establish good habits (but, to establish these good habits in the first place, you'll have to tune in to nutritional information).

(Mostly) Skip the Sweets

At this point you are probably three, four, or maybe even five weeks into making dietary changes. You might even be starting to see some changes in your body. Or not. If you feel like you've been at it a few weeks and your pants are still snug, don't despair! This is a marathon, not a sprint. Remember, the goal is to make one lifestyle change per week. This is not necessarily going to result in rapid weight loss. You need to be patient and keep working on modifications that you think you can sustain for the rest of your life. I know this may seem daunting and not quite fast enough, but it works! Stick with it, and, once you've gotten a handle on your less-than-healthy drinking and snacking habits, take a look at your sweet tooth. It isn't necessary to completely eliminate sweets from your diet, especially if you really enjoy them. However, sweets tend to have fairly little nutritional value and are high in sugar, fat, and calories. Any reduction you can make in the portion or type of sweets you consume is worth your consideration.

When it comes to sweets, there is often a trade-off between quantity and quality. You can have a small portion of Ben & Jerry's ice cream (1/2 cup of vanilla ice cream is 200 calories, 110 of those calories are from fat) or a larger portion of Dryer's vanilla ice cream (3/4 cup is 218 calories, 107 calories from fat) for similar calorie and fat intake. I'd rather have the Ben and Jerry's any day, but the trick then is to watch the portion size—and that can easily become a losing battle. For a while, my husband and I were buying single-serving containers of Ben & Jerry's for dessert (approximately 1/2 cup portions). Then, we decided that just wasn't quite enough to satisfy our sweet tooth, so I started buying pints of ice cream in addition so we could scoop a dollop of ice cream on top of our single-serving portions. Who were we fooling? One day, my husband looked at the portion of ice cream he had prepared himself and laughed. It was clear that we were defeating the purpose of portion control; we had to stick with smaller portions of "the good stuff" or switch what we were eating so that we could enjoy larger portions. This isn't to suggest that you should never indulge in a giant banana split. The trick is to come to terms with the fact that you can eat some sweets regularly, as long as you don't make a habit of going crazy with how much. I mean, if I could, I would eat a pint of Ben & Jerry's every night! I know I'm not the only one; I think it is pretty typical to want to eat a lot of sweets. Indulging in the occasional high-calorie sweet is okay, but frequently overindulging is not a recipe for weight loss and healthy weight management for the long term.

Believe it or not, there are many options for relatively low-calorie (and even low-fat) sweet treats that you can eat on most days. For example, a 1/2 cup portion of Häagen-Dazs raspberry sorbet has 110 calories (and zero grams of fat). This is a healthier option than ice cream, and many find it to be just as tasty. Popsicles, although typically devoid of nutritional value, are tasty and low in calories. Because they are frozen, they take a while to eat, leaving you feeling like you've had a bigger treat than you actually had. For example, Edy's all natural fruit bars have approximately 80 calories and even contain some real fruit. If you want to boost the nutritional value of your sweets, try making smoothies. A blended beverage containing yogurt (try Greek yogurt for additional protein), fruit (purchase large bags of frozen fruit for the best value), nonfat milk, and even a tablespoon of sorbet is a great way to consume some relatively healthy foods in one sweet concoction. I am constantly pushing smoothies on my kids as a way to increase their fruit consumption and satisfy their sweet cravings; smoothies can be a snack, dessert, part of a breakfast, lunch, or dinner. Leftovers get frozen into homemade popsicles for later treats.

I've had women who take part in my research tell me that they were able to successfully change their sweet consumption by reserving sweets for dessert only (cutting out afternoon sweets or breakfasts that were nothing more than sweets). I've also had participants claim that switching to "diet desserts" (e.g., Skinny Cow brand) was an easy fix for them. They still had sweets on many or even most days, but they just made better choices. Some ideas of sweet fixes worth trying are listed in the table below.

SCRUMPTIOUS SWEETS

Dessert	Serving Size	Calories	Fat (g)	Fiber (g)	Protein (g)	Sugar (g)
Angel Food Cake	1 slice (1/12 of cake, 28 g)	72	0.2	0.4	1.7	12
Chocolate-Covered Pretzels	3 (medium size) pretzels (33 g)	150	6	1	2	12
Chocolate-Covered Raisins	1/4 cup (50 g)	211	8.9	1.1	2.2	30
Frozen Strawberry Fruit Bar	1 bar (100 g)	70	0	0.5	0	15
Frozen Yogurt (Flavors Other Than Chocolate)	1/2 cup (87 g)	110.5	3.1	0	2.6	18.7
Fun-Size Snickers	1 bar (15 g)	71	3.6	0.3	1.1	7.6
Fun-Size Butterfinger	1 bar (18 g)	83	3.4	0.4	1	8.3
Vanilla Gelato	1/2 cup (66g)	157	6	2	0	21.6
Gummy Bears	11 bears	100	0	0	2	14
Chocolate Hazelnut Spread	2 tbsp (37 g)	200	11	2	2	20
Hershey's Kisses	9 kisses	200	12	1	3	23
Strawberry Jell-O	1/8 package (2 g)	10	0	0	1	0
Peanut Butter Cookies	2 cookies (30 g)	144	7	0.6	2.8	9.6
Chocolate Pudding	4 oz (108 g)	153	5	0	2.3	18.5
Vanilla Pudding	4 oz (110 g)	143	4.2	0	1.6	18.7
Skinny Cow Salted Caramel Pretzel Ice Cream Bars	1 bar	160	9	2	2	13
Trader Joe's Reduced Guilt Fat-Free Brownies	1/12 of the mix	130	0	1	3	21
Trader Joe's Raspberry Sorbet	1/2 cup	130	0	1	0	25
Twizzler Twists	4 pieces (38 g)	133	0.9	0	1	15.1
Water Ice (a.k.a., Italian Ice)	1 cup (232 g)	122	0	0	0	30
Yogurt-Covered Raisins	1/4 cup	130	5	1	1	19

Note: All nutritional values provided in this table are based on best estimates, but specifics may vary depending on brands of items or exact size of fruits.

> *The biggest seller is cookbooks and the second is diet books—how not to eat what you've just learned how to cook.*
>
> —Andy Rooney

What About Meals?

Remember that weight loss is possible when energy out exceeds the energy in. But how much energy do you really need in the form of food and drinks? It is easiest to reduce nonnutritive caloric intake in the form of drinks, snacks, and sweets, which is why I recommend modifying those habits first. However, some modification to your meals is likely necessary if you want to lose weight and maintain a healthy weight status that you are happy with for the rest of your life.

In general, men can consume around 2,300 calories to maintain their weight, while women can consume around 1,800 calories to maintain their weight.[11] However, these are general estimates that do not take into account people's age, height, current weight, current caloric intake, and activity level. If you are interested in determining the number of calories that you should consume each day to maintain a healthy weight or to lose weight, I recommend you go to the ChooseMyPlate.gov web page and enter your height, weight, and age information. This is where most diet plans and books are incredibly misleading; they typically require specific numbers of calories and specific types of foods that you should eat to lose weight. But they don't take into account individual variations. So, for example, if you are a woman and you currently consume 1,600 calories per day on average, then increasing your caloric intake to 1,800 would lead you to gain weight, not lose it.

For each person, the size and number of calories for each meal is going to be a little bit different depending on his or her current eating and physical activity habits (this is why you started by evaluating your eating and activity habits). However, when pressed, my general recommendation is that men consume 400-calorie breakfasts, 500-calorie lunches, and 900-calorie dinners plus 500 calories worth of snacks, sweets, or beverages that fall outside of primary meals. This amounts to the approximately 2,300 calories per day (400 + 500 + 900 + 500) that men typically require to maintain a healthy weight. Because women's energy needs are lower (which is most certainly one of the greatest injustices in this world!), they may want to use the general guideline of 300 calories for breakfast, 400 calories for lunch, 700 calories for dinner, plus 400 calories for snacks, sweets, or beverages that fall outside of primary meals. This amounts to the approximately 1,800 calories per day (300 + 400 + 700 + 400) that women typically require to maintain a healthy weight. Remember, you must consider this in conjunction with your current habits! If this is an increase in caloric intake, then you will gain rather than lose weight.

To begin losing weight, see my suggestions below for modifying your meals. Keep in mind that you will be best served by modifying your current habits, not necessarily changing them dramatically. If you are not a big breakfast person or find yourself rushed getting ready for your day, then you may eat less in the morning (additional discussion about breakfast can be found in Chapter 7). Forcing yourself to whip up an elaborate breakfast is unlikely to be a reasonable long-term change to your diet. It is essential that you think about the long term and your particular lifestyle and preferences when initiating any dietary or physical activity change.

Breakfast

Breakfast is sometimes called the most important meal of the day, but many people consume little more than large quantities of coffee in the morning. I am not going to condemn coffee consumption; as I mention earlier in this chapter, many coffee drinks are relatively low in calories, and there is research to suggest that caffeine consumption improves mood and attention span.[12] (I'm pretty sure I would not have been able to write this book without coffee!) However, some nutritional food in addition to your cup of joe is highly recommended for the sake of your health, well-being, and even ability to concentrate. To be sure that you actually eat some nutritional food item(s) for breakfast, you need to plan the night before. It is difficult to think straight when groggy, tired, and trying to get out the door in the morning. The manufacturers of packaged breakfast foods know that your mind might not be working at 100 percent and capitalize on it well!

Try including some fruit in your morning meal. Personally, I find a banana a great addition to breakfast—they come in their own organic "wrapper," they can be eaten on the go, and they are high in fiber, potassium, magnesium, vitamin B6, and vitamin C. However, a piece of fruit is unlikely to hold you over for very long. Some sort of more complex carbohydrate is also likely necessary to provide you with the energy you need to start your day. Cereal, oatmeal, toast, or an English muffin can be good choices. Be sure to check the caloric, fiber, and sugar content of these food items (especially for dry cereals, which tend to be high in sugar) before making any particular food a daily habit. A cup of regular Cheerios contains 100 calories, 1 gram of sugar, and 3 grams of fiber (note: this is the nutritional information without milk added—always be careful in reading food labels for little caveats like this). In contrast, a cup of Lucky Charms contains 142 calories, 14 grams of sugar, and 1.6 grams of fiber. Thus, if you choose the healthier cereal, not only will your health benefit, but you can eat more. A reasonable breakfast can consist of a cup of Cheerios with low-fat milk (assuming your portion size really is just a cup, approximately 150 calories), a banana (approximately 100 calories), and a coffee with about as much cream as you like (about 50 calories). Another option is a hard-boiled egg (75 calories), an English muffin (100 calories), a banana (100 calories), and a lighter coffee (minimal cream and calorie-free sweetener). A Greek yogurt (typically higher in protein and lower in calories [approximately 100] than other types of yogurt) or a smoothie that contains fruit, yogurt, and nonfat milk may be a nice part of a breakfast as well (some ingredients can be put in the blender the night before, refrigerated, and then blended in the morning). Remember, once you get to know the nutritional facts concerning your daily morning foods, you should not spend any more time reading the national labels of these foods or thinking about their caloric content.

Eating a satisfying meal in the morning is a good start to eating well throughout the rest of the day. For many people, modifying your breakfast means *adding* healthy foods to this meal, such as a piece of fruit, or switching a relatively unhealthy cereal for one that is both more nutritious and lower in calories and fat. However, there are many breakfast traps that are easy to fall into. For many, junk food for breakfast is fairly typical and not the best way to start your day. Many breakfast foods (e.g., muffins and scones) are really desserts (in terms of their nutritional, caloric, and sugar content) disguised as breakfasts. I love doughnuts, but I know better than to eat them for breakfast. As you evaluate your breakfast habits, be sure that you are honest with yourself, and don't eat a pastry for breakfast just because it is sold at the same place where you pick up your coffee.

Lunch

Most kids like peanut butter and jelly sandwiches for lunch. As a kid, I never really liked them. I actually never really liked most sandwiches. Thus, my nontraditional approach to lunch began a very long time ago. To this day, I don't have "main entrée" for my lunch; instead, I eat an assortment of foods at my desk for lunch: a piece of fruit (or two), a piece of cheese, nuts, vegetables, popcorn. Although some research suggests it is a bad idea to eat while you work, it has been an adaptive approach for my lifestyle.[13] In contrast, you may choose to prepare yourself a sandwich and use lunch as a break in your day. Being mindful of what you eat and enjoying it (i.e., not working while you eat) has its benefits, and many people will ultimately eat *less* if they focus on their meal as opposed to eating while doing something else.[14] Regardless, preparation is necessary if you want to get in the habit of eating a healthy lunch.

Once you've made gradual changes to your beverage, snack, sweets, and breakfast consumption, make an alteration to your lunch. Let's say that you bring or buy a sandwich wherever you are during lunchtime (home, school, work, the mall) and grab a bag of chips to go with it. Instead of chips, have two pieces of fruit. I know, fruit doesn't necessarily taste as good as Cool Ranch Doritos, and fruit perishes, introducing all sorts of planning complications. However, I'm guessing there is *some* sort of fruit that you really like. Maybe something more exotic than the standard apples, bananas, and oranges. How about berries, melon, or mangos? (If you put in a bit of effort you *can* find these fruit options year round. You can even order fruit on the Internet!) Worried about bruising your peach or squishing your berries en route? Nothing a Tupperware container can't handle! If you aren't a fruit person, get in the habit of snacking on veggies during lunch. Supermarkets contain a variety of ready-to-eat veggies (not just carrots), and veggies left over from the previous night's dinner can be a great snack the following day. Make a commitment to put forth the energy to keep stocked up on fruit and veggies that you love to eat.

If you're looking for more calories to easily cut while also improving the health of your lunch, take a look at what's inside your sandwich or on top of your salad. Condiments can ruin any healthy food by adding oil, fat, and sugar. Admittedly, it is the oily, fatty, and sugary goodness that makes a lot of foods taste the way we want them to. I mean, who wants to eat lettuce without salad dressing? As my kids tell me, lettuce just tastes like leaves. It needs a bit of help to become palatable. However, salad dressing and mayonnaise can contain more hidden calories than seems possible in a small serving. Two tablespoons of Caesar salad dressing contains approximately 150 calories. A light Italian salad dressing will contain less than half that. If you really prefer Caesar, try mixing it with some light Italian dressing to "water down" the calories and fat without losing all of the taste. Likewise, about a tablespoon of mayonnaise contains nearly 100 calories. A light mayo may be worth considering instead, at about 35 calories per tablespoon.

If you're thinking, "Did I really buy this book to be told that I should eat light salad dressing? That's pretty obvious!" I agree with you—but that's not really my point. The point of this approach to weight loss and weight management is to make smart, calculated, thoughtful choices about what you eat and establish new healthy habits that you can sustain indefinitely. I could tell you exactly what you should eat for lunch, but if you didn't like my suggestions, you wouldn't stick to my advice. Instead, I want you to think about what you usually eat and modify it to make it a bit healthier. Maybe you like real mayo and don't want to skip having it on your sandwiches. That's okay; find something else to modify. Or, maybe you'll discover that honey mustard (approximately 30 calories a tablespoon and no fat) is pretty darn good and you don't need mayo. Be careful not to be fooled by advertising and labels suggesting that foods are healthy, light, or diet. Read labels closely before establishing new habits. And whatever modification you make to your lunch, ask yourself, "Is this a change that I can make for the rest of my life?"

I surveyed more than a hundred people to see what sorts of healthy options they like to have for lunch. Below is a summary of some of their ideas with approximate calorie information. Keep in mind that these are just ideas. You need to create a custom lunch plan that you find satisfying and enjoyable, or this is not going to work for you long-term.

Dinner

Is this you—eat on the go in the morning, eat relatively healthily during the day, and overindulge at dinner? I'll admit it; this often describes me. Although I find breakfast and lunch nice and necessary, dinner is the meal that I find truly relaxing and enjoyable. I love to sit down with my

LUNCH IDEAS	CALORIE INFORMATION
Fat-free Greek yogurt	120
1/4 cup sliced almonds	+ 150
1 apple	+ 80
1 orange	+ 50
	400
Peanut butter sandwich	
2 pieces of whole wheat bread	200
1 tbsp peanut butter	+ 100
1 banana	+ 100
	400
Trader Joe's (prepackaged) Greek Salad	330
1/2 cup of blueberries	+ 50
	380
2 eggs (scrambled in cooking spray)	150
top with 1/4 cup shredded cheese	+ 100
1 English muffin w/ minimal butter	+ 140
	390
Turkey sandwich	
2 pieces of whole wheat bread	200
3 thin slices of turkey	+ 100
mustard, lettuce, and tomato	+ 30
1 banana	+ 100
	430
Healthy Choice chicken noodle soup (entire can; 2 servings)	180
10 Saltine crackers	+ 120
1 cup of strawberries	+ 90
	390
1 veggie burger	120
1 wheat bun	+180
mustard, tomato, and lettuce	+ 30
1 orange	+ 50
	380

family at the end of the workday and eat and talk—and eat! Sometimes milk is spilled, kids yell at each other, and there is complaining about my food (just because I study food doesn't make me a gourmet cook). Sometimes, dinner is less than a perfect experience, but I still really enjoy a good meal at the end of the workday. On the weekend, a dinner out with friends or a date with my husband can wipe out all the stresses of the workweek. The trick, for me and many other people, is to eat consistently well throughout the day so that dinner doesn't become a gorge-fest. It is important not be too hungry at dinnertime, or poor choices will be made.

What do you usually eat for dinner? Sadly, the "standard American diet" (appropriately, abbreviated SAD) incorporates some of the most unhealthy foods available, and many of them end up on our dinner plates.[15] These avoidable ingestible errors include animal fats, saturated fats, foods low in fiber, highly processed foods, foods low in complex carbohydrates, and sparse amounts of plant-based foods (i.e., fruits and vegetables). If dinner for you consists of a hamburger on a plain bun with mayo and ketchup and a side of French fries, you're dining on several of the SAD favorites: high levels of fat in hamburger meat, a bun devoid of complex carbs and fiber, sugary and fatty condiments, processed and fatty fries. Substituting a chicken breast or a veggie burger could greatly improve upon this meal by cutting out some of the animal fat and calories. Add some lettuce and tomato to your burger and drop the mayo and ketchup. Skip the fries and switch them for some fruit and a side salad. Or at least reduce the portion of fries and try baking them. Homemade fries are cheaper, better for you, and require very little preparation (five minutes to peel and cut potatoes and fifteen to bake in olive oil is not much longer than sticking frozen fries in the oven) and taste wonderful.

Although my intent is not to tell you exactly what to eat and to encourage you to think for yourself about healthy (or at least improved) options for meals, you should incorporate at least one vegetable into each dinner. Even better, throw in some fruit as well. Incorporating some sort of lean protein such as fish, chicken, or beans is ideal. An easy way to boost the nutritional value of a meal is to cut out bread or rolls and include fruit and vegetables instead. Growing up, we always had bread as a side dish. I love bread and would never recommend giving it up, but unless it is a grainy, nutritionally dense bread, it probably is adding little to the healthfulness of your meal. In contrast, just about any fruit or veggie will add not only bulk to your meal but a variety of necessary nutrients. I'm always amazed at the quantity of vegetables my family is able to put away during a dinner (admittedly, my kids help out little in this regard). However, the veggies—whether they be broccoli, string beans, edamame, carrots, or cauliflower—are all relatively low in caloric density, and mass consumption has many benefits with no real drawbacks. The main idea to remember is you need to adopt dietary changes that you can maintain long-term—really, forever. Small one-time changes—like eliminating the side of bread at dinner on Saturday—are unlikely to reduce your pant size, but by skipping the bread basket as a general rule moving forward, you will likely be rocking skinny jeans in a few months, jeans that you continue to rock for years. You see, if you *reduce 200 calories from your diet each day* (or one large bread roll), that's 6,000 calories over a month. Across the year, that would be 72,000 calories, or a reduction of *more than 20 pounds.* Yes, this kind of weight loss can take time, but it isn't painful, and it's weight that will stay off because it is a result of healthy behavior changes. And it won't take you an entire year to feel better. Within a couple of weeks, you will begin to notice that your pants feel a bit loser.

Follow by Example

Even with all that you've learned in this book so far, it can be hard to objectively and honestly evaluate our own food choices. So, let's revisit Julie's food diary, originally presented in Chapter 3. By examining someone else's food choices and thinking about improvements that she can make to her eating habits, you may be inspired to make similar choices for your own beverages, snacks, sweets, and meals.

II

Julie's Food Diary

TIME	FOOD/DRINKS CONSUMED/ PHYSICAL ACTIVITIES	REFLECTION/MOOD
6am		
7am	Coffee w/ 2 splenda and ¼ cup of half and half Oatmeal (package; 180 cal)	Fine, tired
8am		
9am	Banana	More awake, fine
10am		
11am		
12pm	Ham sandwich (2 pieces of wheat bread, 2 slices of ham, mustard, lettuce); water	Good
1pm		
2pm	Bag of Doritos chips (cool ranch flavor); Diet Coke	Guilty about chips, but they tasted good
3pm	Walked for 30 minutes on treadmill	Great while walking; relaxed
4pm	Apple dipped in peanut butter (1 tablespoon); water	Good
5pm		
6pm	2 cups pasta w/ pesto sauce. 1 small grilled chicken breast (about 5 in by 4 in). 1 cup of carrots. 1 glass of white wine.	Fine
7pm		
8pm		
9pm	Ben and Jerry's ice cream, chocolate chip cookie dough flavor (1 cup)	Tired
10pm		
11pm		
12 midnight		
1am		

Consisting of primarily water, coffee, and Diet Coke, there isn't a lot of room for improvement in Julie's beverage consumption. A Diet Coke may not be the best choice for health, but it is unlikely to make her gain weight. Water is a better option but may not provide the midday "pick me up" desired. Julie could try to cut out her glass of wine with dinner to drop approximately 120 nonnutritive calories from her diet. Milk is a great addition to a dinner, with calcium, vitamin D, and other nutritional benefits.

Next, let's evaluate her snack consumption. Julie had a banana for a morning snack, which is a great option, as is the apple and peanut butter for her afternoon snack. However, a bag of Doritos is not a good daily snack habit. Popcorn, fruit, or some of the other options in the table provided earlier in this chapter are all healthier alternatives. A piece of fruit in the afternoon may lead to a lighter dinner later, so skipping the snack is not the idea—swapping it for something healthier is the way to go.

Julie's sweet consumption consisted of Ben & Jerry's ice cream for dessert—just the sort of dessert I like to indulge in as well. Remember, the goal is not necessarily to eliminate all sweets. However, she may want to consider reducing the portion size or having sorbet some evenings instead of ice cream (sorbet is lower in fat and calories). A small serving of vanilla ice cream with some raspberries or other fruit (even frozen fruit) would provide more nutritional value than just ice cream, but dessert isn't necessarily about obtaining the vitamins, minerals, or nutrients needed. Food should be enjoyed, and it should not feel like a chore!

Julie's breakfast is fairly typical and a reasonable choice. However, instant oatmeal can hide a lot of sugar, and another cereal or toast option may ultimately be healthier. Adding fruit to breakfast is also worth considering. Her lunch and dinner present more opportunity for improvement. Julie's ham sandwich for lunch is not a bad idea—especially if it is homemade (portion sizes are inevitably larger when you eat out, so packing lunch at home to bring with you is always a good idea). Selecting a whole grain wheat bread that is nutritionally dense is important, as is limiting condiment use. Further, adding additional veggies—tomato, pickles, peppers—would boost the health value of this sort of sandwich. Julie's dinner choices of chicken and carrots are excellent. The pasta may be less than optimal. Unless the pasta is whole grain, it likely provides little nutritional benefit, and the pesto sauce may provide substantial caloric and fat content. So, reducing the pasta to 1 cup and adding another vegetable would be one way to improve this meal.

It is obvious that Julie is already thoughtful about what she eats and spends some time and energy planning and making her meals (e.g., bringing a banana as a snack in the morning). The healthy modifications I've suggested to Julie's diet are not extreme; they are actually fairly subtle. However, if she changed her daily eating habits according to my recommendations, she would reduce her intake by approximately 400 calories per day. If these small changes are sustained, she will lose weight and feel better. In fact, if changes like the ones I suggested are maintained across a year, she would lose approximately forty pounds! Notice that she didn't note feeling particularly good when she ate chips or ice cream. Like all of us, Julie's dietary habits should be viewed as a work in progress. The goal is to modify what you already eat, change your habits gradually, and become more thoughtful about your choices. The idea isn't to embark on an extreme fast or abandon any food group or favored food item. The idea is to make practical, realistic changes across time that will improve your health, reduce your weight, and make you feel good physically and psychologically. Don't make this harder than it has to be. Remember, food is fun.

- Modifying what you eat bite by bite is the best way to lose weight over the long haul.
- Start by evaluating and changing—in this order—beverages, snacks, desserts, and then meals.
- This phase brings you back to the basics of healthy eating and is the opposite of what most diet plans propose (which usually entails severe restriction at the start of a diet and then adding back other foods across time); this smart way of approaching weight loss makes all the difference if you plan to lose weight and keep it off!

STAY
SMART

Get Moving

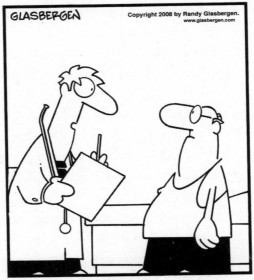

GLASBERGEN

Copyright 2008 by Randy Glasbergen.
www.glasbergen.com

"What fits your busy schedule better, exercising one hour a day or being dead 24 hours a day?"

It's easier to wake up each morning and work out than it is to look in the mirror each day and not like what you see.

Jayne Cox, specialist women's coach

About a year before my husband turned forty, he began to pay more attention to what he ate, and he started exercising. After nearly fifteen years of living with me (for all but a couple of which he seemed to go out of his way to *avoid* exercise), he finally revamped his health habits. What can I say, like most men, my husband can be stubborn, but after the birth of our second child he decided it was time to get healthy and live a long life! When this resulted in weight loss and people asked him about it, he would always say, "Oh, I just started running." I think that he didn't want to explain his weight loss in terms of something that sounded like a diet, and it was far more macho to talk about fitness. For a couple of years now, he has exercised nearly every day. This is a guy who used to say things like, "Why run when you can drive?" My proud couch potato is in the best shape he has ever been in (he slowly lost forty pounds across eight months and has kept it off for years). I love that I now have another person I can run with, and I find him an interesting and inspirational case of how even the most reluctant exerciser can become physically fit. This isn't to say that this just happened overnight. In fact, he very gradually and somewhat reluctantly began to exercise. But if he can, anyone can!

Physical fitness is an important component of the weight management equation. You cannot think about weight loss and maintaining a healthy weight without incorporating some form of physical activity into your regular routine. Having said that, just beginning an exercise regimen is an unlikely means of achieving weight loss. It is important to be thoughtful about *both* what you eat and your physical activity. One helps the other. Hopefully, you've kept track of your physical activities while you were recording your food intake. If you are like most Americans, there isn't much to keep track of. Maybe you've been working toward participating in regular physical activity—whether that is once a week or every day of the week. Perhaps you don't have the time, or you simply aren't motivated. Working exercise into our regular routines is not a simple thing to do. This chapter will teach you how to become

In this chapter you will learn . . .
- The important physical and psychological benefits of regular physical activity
- How becoming and staying physically active will help you lose weight and keep it off for the long haul
- Ideas to help get you started on a new (or enhanced) exercise routine and stay inspired for years to come

smart when it comes to exercise, because no thoughtful approach to weight loss and management can neglect the importance of moving your body!

Exercise is one of the best ways in preventing the rapid growth of obesity in America.

—**Lee Haney, body builder, Mr. Olympia**

An Inactive America

Some days, I wake up early to exercise, and I can't help but wonder, "Why am I doing this?" I know that the majority of Americans are not exercising—or not exercising very much. In fact, less than half of the US population engages in enough exercise to stay healthy. One out of every three Americans gets no physical activity at all! Men are more likely to be physically active than women, but most men and women should exercise more than they do. Perhaps more troubling, almost half of US children do not participate in the necessary amount of exercise to benefit their health.[1] Even among teenagers—who always seem on the go— only two out of every ten are getting the recommended amount of exercise. Crazy, huh? The fact that only three out of every ten teens have some sort of daily school-based physical education is an obvious contributor to these low rates of physical activity.[2]

There are regional differences in those who exercise in the United States, with individuals residing on the West Coast, Colorado, Minnesota, and parts of the Northeast being most likely to be active. My initial thought was to attribute these regional differences to weather (my experience has taught me that it is easier to go for a run in the winter in California than in Pennsylvania); however, the most active states have a range of different climates. The states with the lowest rates of activity (or, as it is often described, the highest rates of "leisure time physical inactivity") are in the South. In fact, if you compare the map below of physical inactivity rates in the United States to the map depicting obesity rates in Chapter 10, you'll see some obvious similarities.[3]

Stop the Screen Insanity

Obviously, I'm going to encourage you to be more active. However, it is necessary to first consider your *inactivity*—in other words, your sedentary behaviors. Modern advances have made it possible to be incredibly sedentary. This is a dramatic switch from the state of affairs a couple hundred of years ago. Not too long ago, heavy people were regarded as attractive because fat was an indicator of wealth. It was a luxury to not have to be physically active in the pursuit of food and to have the resources to acquire enough food to allow you to be round.[4] Nowadays, getting food is pretty effortless for most of us in the industrialized world. Getting exercise requires a great deal more effort.

One of the greatest detractors from exercise time is "screen time." A recent report based on a survey of kids eight to eighteen years of age indicates that in half of their homes TV is left on "most of the time." Add in video games, computers, iPads, and other sources of screens, and kids spend more than seven hours per day (fifty-three hours per week) sitting

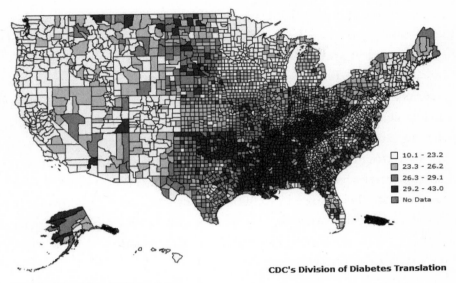

CDC's Division of Diabetes Translation

Leisure-Time Physical Inactivity

and watching instead of running around. Adults are lucky if they suck up only seven hours of screen time *each day*. With jobs increasingly requiring connecting to others around the world electronically, adults' screen time just using computers tends to exceed children's. Such use of technology is why, over the past fifty years, most adults found themselves sitting down on the job. Translation: we burn 150 fewer calories per day on average than the more active working generation that came before us. Stay-at-home parents are also getting less physical activity and more screen time than they once did. Stay-at-homers burn approximately 360 fewer calories per day in the twenty-first century than they did in the 1960s.[5]

All of this screen time is linked with obesity in direct and indirect ways. If you're sitting watching TV, you aren't exercising, and you are more likely to be eating. It's a double whammy. Less physical activity and more snacking (usually on high-calorie nonnutritive foods) is a quick way to pack on extra pounds. What is even more discouraging is that research has found that not only do people eat while engaging in screen time; they eat foods that are heavily advertised—on those very screens![6]

Although it sounds simple, setting screen-time limits really does reduce how much time people engage in sedentary activities. Maybe this means establishing personal or family rules like no TV in the morning before work or school or no TV while in bed at night, or you could even try no eating in front of the TV (that may help preserve your sofa as well). Setting limits on how many hours per day people have access to screens is very helpful and will free up time for physical activity. One recent study that followed 240,000 adults over 8.5 years found that high levels of television consumption was associated with higher mortality rates. If nothing else, consider exercising while watching TV (or whatever screen you prefer).

Just Get Moving!

So, now that you have the TV off, let's talk about getting moving. There are many different ways to exercise and be physically active. You may have noticed that I use the terms "physical activity" and "exercise" interchangeably. I'm sure scholars who make a career of studying these issues will scoff that I'm not differentiating between them. According to these scientists, physical activity refers to any, well, physical activity. Anything that gets you moving, your muscles working, and your heart beating a little faster is physical activity. You might work up a sweat gardening, or you feel out of breath when chasing after your toddler. Maybe, you feel tired after cleaning your house or climbing the stairs at work. All of this constitutes physical activity.

Exercise, in contrast, is typically used to describe physical activity that is more purposeful, like going to the gym. You may start an exercise regimen to get in shape or to lose weight. If you are training for a race or an event, then you are exercising. In other words, exercise is always a physical activity, but all physical activities are not exercise. Usually exercise is more intense than physical activity. Walking around the mall as you shop or having sex with a partner (usually) qualifies as physical activity, but I know few people who would categorize these activities as exercise. Although the terms are distinct, I intentionally blur this difference throughout this chapter. I do this for a reason: I don't want you to think of exercise as something that always has to be planned or purposeful. I want you to focus on being active as much as possible, no matter how, when, or why. In terms of both health and weight loss, it is not important what we call it. Although purposeful exercise is an efficient technique to maintain weight loss, daily physical activity (i.e., not just sitting on the couch or in an office all day) is also important. In other words, just move! It is essential that you not just take in energy (in the form of calories) but that you also expend some of this energy through movement on a regular basis.[7]

The When-You-Have-Time-For-It Workout

So, how much time will it take you to actually exercise? I understand that you already have a full life. You probably have a job (or jobs). Maybe you are in school. You most likely have responsibilities to other people, whether they are your children, coworkers, friends, or your aging parents. Taking time to exercise is often viewed as a luxury that most people cannot afford. But what if I were to tell you that just thirty-minute workouts would do the trick? Can you afford that?

For exercise to offer you real fitness and health benefits, adults need 150 minutes (that's two and a half hours) of exercise a week.[8] Adults should also participate in both aerobic activity (brisk walking, jogging, or running) as well as muscle-strengthening activities (push-ups, sit-ups). Children should be physically active for approximately an hour a day. This is important not only for weight management but for developmental purposes. For example, exercise helps to strengthen growing bones. Michelle Obama knows this, and her Let's Move campaign has a goal of getting all kids moving for sixty minutes per day.[9] With the aim of including 50,000 schools and with corporate sponsors like Nike investing $50 million to support this goal, we can only hope that this generation of kids spends more time in gym class than they do in doctors' offices.

To get 2.5 hours of exercise a week, you'd need to exercise for thirty minutes, five days a week. If this feels like more of a time commitment than you're willing or able to make, don't sweat it—you don't have to do it all now. Just as it is with adopting a smarter approach to healthy eating, the smart approach to making changes to your physical activities is also gradual, realistic, and moderate. If you don't have thirty minutes, five days a week, maybe you have thirty minutes once a week? Maybe you have time for a sixty-minute exercise class each weekend? Hear this now: *any physical activity is better than no physical activity.* Further, it is entirely possible that committing to even moderate amounts of exercise per week may inspire you to try to do more. Some experts recommend trying three ten-minute walks a day, five days a week.[10] This may be a walk to work, walking your kids to and from the park, walking the dog in the morning and afternoon, or taking a ten-minute walk during your lunch hour. Although this may seem like a lot of walks to keep track of, with a bit of discipline, you can reach 2.5 hours per week without necessarily feeling like you are "exercising."[11] The opposite approach is also recommended by some: "vigorous intensity activity" for twenty minutes, three days per week, may have the same advantages as does more exercise of lower intensity.[12] Further, some recent research suggests that four workouts per week may be better than six and that your body may burn calories more efficiently if you exercise a moderate amount per week and *not* every day.[13]

Although there may be no obvious, clear agreement about how much to exercise, for how many days per week, and at what intensity, any physical activity is better than no physical activity. We will not all be marathon runners, and we will not all develop six-packs. However, we do want to be able to walk up a flight of stairs without feeling winded. The more we move, the better off our health and the looser our pants.

MEGAN'S *Story*

I joined CrossFit over two years ago, but it took me almost a year to really start going regularly. Now, I can honestly say it has been one of the best additions to my life. I had been trying for years after high school to find some form of exercise that kept me interested and made me want to do it. That's what CrossFit does for me. Initially, I went about once a week. Then something just clicked, and I started going consistently three times a week. I think I realized how much happier I was after finishing a CrossFit class, and that's what really changed my behavior. I gradually started increasing the number of days that I attend classes, and I now go five or six days a week.

I've also found that there is a relationship between exercise and eating right. I think finally realizing that I'm never going to lose the weight I want to or "feel better" by just doing one or the other was key. I decided I had to do both. I have finally gotten the exercise portion where I want it to be, and now I'm focusing more attention on eating better. Because I think of CrossFit as more of an everyday thing in my life now, I no longer have to force myself to do it. It's not a chore; it's just something that I do as a part of my daily routine.

~Megan, AGE TWENTY-FOUR, STUDENT

How Much Will This Help Me Lose Weight?

How much exercise will actually help you to lose weight depends on how much you exercise (minutes or hours), how vigorously, and how often (days per week). In the past couple of years, I've gone from running approximately fifteen miles per week to running more than twenty, plus swimming for up to a couple of hours per week. How much weight have I lost? None—nada—zero pounds! In increasing my exercise regimen, I was not trying to lose weight; my goals have been fitness, health, and stress management. But why haven't I lost weight? Simple: the more I exercise, the more I eat; exercising can make you hungry! I share this personal example with you not to discourage you but to help you understand that exercise should be part of a healthy approach to weight management, but exercise alone is not enough for long-term weight loss. If you are aiming to *lose* weight, then you need to keep your eating habits stable (or reduce your intake) while you *increase* your activity.

If you maintain the same eating habits but exercise for just fifteen minutes per day (burning approximately 100 calories per day), you will not notice a rapid change in your weight. However, if you maintain this daily exercise routine, you will burn about 36,500 calories in a year—or lose about ten pounds. Not bad for fifteen minutes! Most exercise equipment at a gym will provide you with approximate estimates of calories burned. (Beware: these are only estimates!) So if you are currently not exercising at all and you start to exercise regularly, you can monitor the energy expended in relation to the energy (calorie) intake. But don't get too hung up on the numbers. Weight loss and weight management should not be a never-ending math problem! Most importantly, once you have your exercise and eating habits established, you should never focus on the numbers—don't burn calories so that you can eat more! The trick is to be active and not to eat more.

The bottom line is that exercise can absolutely help you lose weight, but you also have to watch what you eat. Sorry, exercise isn't a free pass to the buffet line, but chew on this: people who exercise regularly tend to feel more invested in eating well and more committed to their health. In other words, the more you exercise, the more likely you will *want* to eat smarter. In fact, going to the gym or on regular walks will likely encourage you to crave healthier foods. Imagine that! And the more you regularly exercise and eat smarter, the easier it will be to maintain a svelte figure. It is easier to have that big piece of chocolate cake at that party and not experience any weight gain if you are regularly burning off some calories. If you commit yourself to changing your lifestyle, losing weight, and thinking long-term about weight management, you'll soon see the benefits of adding physical activity to your weekly routine.

Another good reducing exercise consists in placing both hands against the table edge and pushing back.

—Robert Quillen, writer

Work Out Your Whole Body

Physical activity has benefits far greater than merely helping you lose weight or maintain a desired weight. Physical activity is associated with improved physical and mental health. For example, individuals who exercise regularly are less likely to experience heart disease, stroke, and some cancers.[14] A study recently published in the prestigious *British Medical Journal* even found that a structured exercise program maintains your cardiovascular health better than prescription drugs.[15] Exercise also helps prevent high blood pressure, high cholesterol, and type 2 diabetes.[16] It can aid in digestion after a meal, strengthen your bones, and reduce your likelihood of developing osteoporosis.[17] Exercise improves sleep habits over time and is even thought to have benefits at the level of our DNA.[18] Perhaps most importantly, people who exercise regularly live longer than people who don't.[19]

If the above health benefits don't motivate you and you happen to possess a Y chromosome, then a new study linking physical activity to sperm count may inspire you.[20] Men who engage in regular physical activity have 73 percent higher sperm counts than men who are less active. Higher sperm count typically means higher fertility. It seems that when a man is more physically fit, his body responds by being better prepared to produce babies (after all, it wouldn't be adaptive for couch potatoes to reproduce as easily as their physically fit peers—right?).

Perhaps you expected me to remind you of the physical benefits of exercise, but did you know that moving your body can actually benefit your psychological health as well? Maybe you've heard people talk about a "runner's high" or feeling "uplifted" as a result of exercise. It turns out that there is something to this; people who exercise regularly are less likely to be depressed than those sitting on couches all day.[21] Exercise also alleviates anxiety and improves mood. There are both biological and psychological reasons for the links between exercise and psychological health. Exercise affects brain functioning by releasing "feel-good brain chemicals" (neurotransmitters and endorphins) that improve mood. Exercise also reduces the immune system chemicals that can negatively impact mood. Even the increase in body temperature following exercise is thought to have a calming effect that indirectly improves your mood.

On a more psychological level, exercise is a healthy distraction from negative thoughts or experiences. I love swimming because no one can bother me while my head is under water and I can't hear anything! Exercise is a healthy coping mechanism. When we feel sad or anxious, it may be tempting to grab a beer or a glass of wine, but going on a walk or run is going to make you feel better. Even children experience the stress-reducing benefits of exercise: children who are regularly physically active have healthier hormonal responses to stressful situations than children who are not as active.[22]

Exercise also increases self-esteem, especially if it provides you with an opportunity to set goals for yourself and then reach them. Because exercise facilitates weight loss, it indirectly helps you feel better about your physical appearance as well. Finally, exercise provides an opportunity for social interaction. I find running with friends much more fun than running alone. I can't say that I'd schedule thirty minutes to catch up with friends on a regular basis (especially not at 6 a.m.!); however, when I run with a friend, not only do I get exercise, but my running partners and I have talked about everything from where we get our groceries to anything and everything about our children to whether God really exists (not necessarily during the same run!). I'm pretty sure all of this random conversation provides about as much psychological benefit as a good therapist would, and it is a lot cheaper![23]

Just Not Pumped?

Newton's first law of motion is "A body remains at rest unless acted upon by an external force." In addition to explaining the motion of heavenly bodies, this law provides an analogy for why many people have trouble starting an exercise program. If your body has been at rest for years, it might feel like an impossible task to get yourself motived to move. So, how can you get yourself pumped up to start exercising if you're lacking the motivation needed to establish an exercise regimen? The secret, like with food changes, is to start out slow. One good place to start is by making modifications to your daily routine. Below is a list of some of the activities you might want to make part of your daily habits. As you'll see, being active doesn't have to involve a gym; being active can involve minor modification to your daily routines.

Ten Things You Can Do Today to Increase Your Physical Activity

1. Take the stairs, skip the elevator.
2. Park far away and walk five minutes to your destination.
3. When you go to check your mail, grab it and walk around the block while you look at it.
4. Do a household chore that you've been avoiding—vacuum, clean out a closet, or wash some windows.

5. Carry your groceries, packages, or small children instead of using a cart, carrier, or stroller.
6. Do twenty sit-ups and twenty push-ups while you watch TV. Do a second set if that goes well.
7. Take a break from work or other responsibilities and take a ten-minute walk while listening to music or an audio book.
8. Wash your car by hand.
9. Work in your garden, pull weeds, plant flowers, or mow the lawn.
10. Dance to music while you study, do the dishes, or play with your kids.

These are all easy, quick things that can have a gradual, significant impact on your health and fitness. In fact, if you do a few of these things each day, you are likely to burn about 100 or more extra calories. Once you start with these minor changes to your activity level, you will notice that you will be more motivated to increase your exercise level. However, remember to keep it slow—no signing up for the Boston Marathon yet!

Of course, some people enjoy the actual act of exercising. Some days I understand this. Many days I don't. I like how I feel when I'm *done* exercising, but I often find the process less than fun. Somehow, I'm still pretty addicted to exercise. Some research suggests that encouraging yourself while you exercise can be motivating. It may sound a bit crazy, but telling yourself you are not tired or engaging in what researchers call "motivational self-talk" (i.e., thinking to yourself, "This feels good," or, "I'm not tired yet") can keep you exercising longer.[24] For me, one of the tricks is to keep myself entertained. I listen to music, I listen to books, and I talk with other people. It seems I'm not alone: folks I see at my gym have all kinds of cool devices—phones, iPads, Kindles—that they bring to the gym with them. There are apps that may help as well (some of which I discuss in Chapter 3). A new app for the iPhone called Cruise Control allows people to "coordinate their pacing with their playlists."[25] Music can help you to walk, run, or pedal faster. On some days, it even keeps me exercising a bit longer because I like the song that I'm listening to.

Taking a walk or riding a stationary bike is a great place to begin or add to your exercise routine. I know people who bring their iPad to the gym and watch TV shows or movies while they ride. A bit of planning to download a video ahead of time, and thirty minutes on a bike can go pretty fast (that's just one TV show). I have a neighbor who has started to get up an hour earlier each morning to walk the indoor track at the gym. He says that he listens to the *New York Times* podcasts in the morning and just walks, and then he gets ready for work at the gym. His routine is relaxing, informative, and a healthy way to start the day.

If biking, running, or walking holds no appeal for you, consider what it is you really like to do. I'm convinced that everyone can find some sort of physical activity that they enjoy. Maybe it is playing a team sport, dancing, or stair racing. Yes, stair racing is a sport growing in popularity, and I have no doubt that it is an intense (and fast!) way to get in some exercise. So if you don't have a lot of time, try running up and down stairs in your office building for fifteen minutes before you leave work. Before you know it, you might become one of the thousands of people racing to the top of the Empire State Building each year for the annual Empire State Building Run Up (that's eighty-six flights of stairs!).[26]

If you never hope to run to the top of the Empire State Building, then exercise classes might be a great way to socialize and exercise at the same time. The fact that there is a set time and location can be helpful. Setting goals, such as "I'm going to Zumba at 6 p.m. after work" can be very motivating. However, if you are currently out of shape or don't know the routines presented in a class, it is easy to feel discouraged. Fortunately, some smart entrepreneurs appreciate the importance of feeling comfortable in a fitness environment, even if you are not (yet) "fit." Fitness centers are popping up that cater to the reluctant or inexperienced exerciser. They aim to make users feel comfortable and motivated to exercise, even though they may not feel like they know quite what they are doing. If this sort of an environment sounds better to you than being in a gym full of sweaty guys in tight tank tops with bulging biceps, do a web search for options in your area or check out www.fit -journey.com for one woman's guide for new gym-goers.[27]

SAMANTHA'S *Story*

I am a forty-two-year-old working mom, so I don't have a lot of free time to fit in exercise. But, as I get older, I realize that I need to exercise to stay healthy and be around for my family as long as I possibly can. I know that grand weight loss won't likely come from exercise, which is why I watch what I eat. But I know that exercising is the key to staying fit and active as I age. It will help keep my heart healthy and help me retain my flexibility.

The most important thing for me was to find the RIGHT exercise. I hate the one-size-fits-all methods where the trainers tell you to run so many miles a week or go to the gym and do this or that circuit. That might work for some. But it is not for me. I need to love what I am doing, or I won't keep doing it. I need to do activities that trick me into forgetting that I am exercising. This is why I Jazzercise three times per week, minimum.

I love to dance, and the routines challenge both my body and by brain. I leave every class covered in sweat with a smile on my face. If I have to miss class because of my schedule, I really do *miss* it. I can't wait until I can get back out there again and dance around the studio. If you hate your workout and dread it, you won't keep doing it for long. I always tell my friends that they need to find something they love to do and stick with it. I just met two women at my Jazzercise studio who have been coming to classes for thirty-seven and twenty-five years. Now that tells you something. They wouldn't keep coming back if it weren't fun!!

~Samantha, AGE FORTY-TWO, CONSULTANT

Let Other People Help You

As you gradually work to incorporate more physical activity into your life, don't feel like you have to go it alone. One of the best ways to change your habits—any sort of habit—is to solicit help. Tell people you are starting an exercise regimen, and ask them to check in with you about your progress. Tell your mom or best friend that each time you talk to her, you want her to ask you how exercising is going. Having this sense of "responsibility" to others can be very powerful. No one wants to admit that they've given up on a goal that is important to them. It also costs nothing for people who care about you to encourage you or make it easier for you to maintain an exercise regimen.

My husband and I often make deals with each other to make it possible for us to both exercise regularly. For a while, I put our kids to bed so that he'd feel motivated to go to the gym. Anyone with toddlers knows that bedtime is not the most fun time of day. Baths need to be taken and stories need to be read. "Escaping" that part of the day to be alone, on an exercise bike, with some music proved to be a pretty powerful incentive. Often, my husband gets our kids fed and dressed in the morning so that I can go running. Although we all love our kids, all parents know that scheduling our lives to maintain demanding jobs, be good parents, and focus on our own health requires strategic planning and help!

Perhaps one of the best ways to maintain an exercise regimen is to find a person (or people) to exercise with. Meet a friend at an exercise class or for a walk once or twice a week. If you can't find someone you already know to exercise with, then ask people you know less well. Ask an acquaintance or a work colleague if he or she would be interested in taking a class or checking out a new fitness center. I've been pleasantly surprised at how receptive people are to the idea of collaborating to achieve fitness goals. Most people appreciate that exercising regularly is challenging and welcome the idea of having someone help them get in better shape. I've actually become good friends with other women because we decided to exercise together; they have tremendously enriched my life besides just helping me to stick with an exercise regimen.

Technology can also be helpful if you want to connect with workout partners. For example, at Rutgers University, there is a program recently developed called Workout with Me that allows students to connect with others via Facebook and Twitter and encourage others to meet them at the campus gym.[28] Students register for the group on the web and can post their workout plans, especially when they don't have anyone to exercise with and would like someone to join them. The aim of the program is for students to encourage each other to work out and to have fun socializing while they do it. There's no reason those of us who have left our college days behind can't also use Facebook, Twitter, or simply texting to try to find workout partners and to encourage those we care about to meet their fitness goals, whether those goals be exercising two times a week or training for a triathlon.

Take It Outdoors

Maybe you feel claustrophobic in a gym, and the full length mirrors are nothing but a depressing reminder of how far you are from your fitness and weight goals. Well, there's some good news for you. Evidence is accumulating that people exercise more regularly and for longer when they exercise outdoors.[29] They also work their muscles differently and expend more energy when exercising outdoors versus on a treadmill or stationary bike. There's even evidence that exercising outdoors lowers your stress hormones while the sunlight boosts your mood. It's also free—no gym membership fees—plus, there's no awkwardness about trying to figure out how to use equipment, no strangers staring at you trying to wear spandex. The only downside is the weather. If it is too hot or too cold, it is hard to exercise outdoors. There is clothing designed for exercise in all terrains and climates, which helps. There is equipment made specifically for exercising outdoors when it is dark. I have accumulated a fair amount of this equipment in recent years and am grateful for it. I'm sure some people think that I am crazy when I go for a run in the snow, with a headlamp and a reflective vest (my kids love to tease me about this look). However, I just tell them that they'll be glad their mom kept her bum moving and worked to maintain her health when they don't have to take care of me later in life.

This isn't to say that the climate can't create challenges for even the most dedicated exerciser. And I don't mind admitting that there are those who are much more motivated than I am and who have accomplished amazing athletic feats I don't ever anticipate accomplishing. However, it can be useful to turn to professional athletes for motivation. Sometimes, watching the pros leaves me truly amazed at what the human body is capable of. It makes me want to get my body working to its fullest potential.

An Interview with Tara Lipinski, Figure Skater, Olympic Gold Medalist, and Sports Commentator

Tara Lipinski became a household name in 1998 when, at fifteen, she became the youngest figure skater to win a gold medal in the winter Olympics. She began skating at age six and ended her competitive career not long after the Olympics, turning to professional skating and touring. Today, she has a fulfilling career as a sports commentator for ice skating with Universal Sports and was a commentator for the winter Olympics in 2014. I interviewed Tara in the process of writing this book because her personal story is inspirational and she provides a great role model for all of us trying to get in shape and stay in shape. Excerpts from this interview are below.

CM: What sort of advice can you offer the average person about how to stay physically active?

TL: Now that I'm not training for competition, I work out and am active for myself and how it makes me feel. Sometimes it is easier to stay motivated than other times, and I'll go through phases when I don't work out regularly. However, I always get back to exercising because I feel so healthy and fit after a good workout. It can take a week or two to establish exercise habits again, but, once you start to feel good from exercising, that feeling is what keeps you going. Exercise can really make you feel more alive— you just have to get in the habit. I guess my advice is that you just have to stick with it—give it some time, and you'll see and feel the results of exercising. It is important to set your mind to goals that are important to you. Physical activity can make you feel accomplished and fit—it is easy to become addicted to that feeling.

CM: When you were competing, how were you able to stay motivated to stick with such long hours of training?

TL: It became such a routine. I always had new goals and new things to work on. Ice skating is a very physical sport and I was always motivated to get ready for competitions.

CM: You experienced some hip injuries during your career. Do you have any words of wisdom about how to stay active, healthy, and avoid injury?

TL: I think it is important to get to know your body and get to know what feels good to you. I think I learned when I was really young what my body can handle and what I enjoy. I also learned that there is "good pain" that you can work through and pain and injury that you need to be careful about and address.

CM: As an athlete, how did you think about fitness, health, and nutrition? Given the media attention you received as a young woman, were you ever concerned about your weight?

TL: Skating is an aesthetic sport, but it is also an athletic sport, and I had to be strong and muscular to do the sport well. I grew up wanting to be strong; I knew that I couldn't be rail thin if I was going to be successful. After my competitive career ended, I worked a bit with a nutritionist to help me maintain healthy eating habits conducive to maintaining my professional career, but my focus has always been on fitness, strength, and health. *I have never "dieted."*

Slow and Steady Wins the Race

As you incorporate exercise into your life and find people to help you maintain your new habits, remember that changing your exercise patterns should be a gradual process. Take it easy and give yourself a break (or you might actually break something). Patience is key. You want to develop habits that you will keep *for the rest of your life*. Further, trying to do too much at once is usually overwhelming and will keep you from doing anything at all. You have to somewhat enjoy or find some value in your exercise habits for them to be sustainable. You don't have to love the actual exercise, but maybe you enjoy the alone time. Maybe you enjoy meeting a friend and seeing him or her once a week. You may just like how you feel after exercising, and that may prove motivating.

Once you review your eating and activity logs, assess the extent to which you are already active and the days that you may be able to work in additional activity. Unfortunately, for many people, exercising regularly means waking up earlier. You should not give up on the necessary amount of sleep (for most adults, seven-plus hours is necessary for not only health but also for weight management).[30] However, you may need to go to bed earlier or cut out thirty minutes of inactive TV time to squeeze in thirty minutes of active time.

If you don't currently exercise at all and you aren't particularly excited to, then start with just becoming more physically active during your day. Next, try adding two thirty-minute episodes of exercise per week. Walk in your neighborhood, walk on a treadmill, or ride an exercise bike. Start easy and see how it goes. If you miss one of your two days of exercise, try to exercise for sixty minutes once that week. After a few weeks, maybe you'll be ready to up the ante a bit. If so, then try jogging for a few minutes instead of only walking. Or raise the level of intensity on your exercise bike. Pick something that you can see yourself continuing to do and that you find relaxing, fun, or feasible with your schedule.

Start your new or enhanced exercise regimen gradually, but consider setting some goals for the next few months. Sign up for a 5K walk, or plan to be able to work up to a certain amount of time on the elliptical machine. Exercise regularly with these goals in mind if you find this motivating. When my children were younger, I could not exercise more than twice a week. There was no way for me to squeeze anything else in (and this was after a few year's hiatus from any activity when I had babies who were up for large portions of the night). After a year or so with this routine, I added a third day per week. The following year, I added a fourth day. It's taken me more than three years, but I'm probably now in the best shape I've ever been in in my life. This is not to say that most people should require three or four years to establish an exercise regimen that they are happy with. I would hope that most people's schedules provide a bit of flexibility and that starting with two or three days per week of at least twenty to thirty minutes of exercise is possible. However, if this is a very long-term "project" for you, that's also okay.

The main thing to remember is to be as active as you can as much as you can without making it a stressful addition to your schedule. Being disciplined is good, but making exercise fun and sustainable is also essential. You don't have to run marathons or spend a great deal of time exercising each week to reap some benefits (both psychological and physical). You should not feel like a failure if you never increase your exercise schedule beyond a couple of outings to the gym per week. Always keep your focus on establishing habits that work for you and are conducive to maintaining your health.

The important thing is not to catch something . . . the important thing is moving.

—Kilian Jornet Burgada, called the most dominating endurance athlete of his generation

---

The Bottom Line

If I had to pick one change for people to make in the name of weight loss, changing their eating habits is easily my choice. It is easier to eat fewer calories than it is to burn off calories. However, there are plenty of changes you can and should make—starting today—to increase your physical activity. Exercise is a great supplement to eating well if your goal is weight loss or weight management over the long term. Losing weight isn't about just looking better but becoming healthier and hopefully even living longer because you take good care of yourself.

Here's one final thought: you may actually like exercising. I remember telling my husband years ago that I felt sorry for him because he didn't exercise and he didn't know how amazing it could feel to do a great workout. It took him more than a decade of watching me exercise before he decided to really give it a try. Now, he swears he'll never go back.

- Exercise has tremendous benefits for your physical and psychological health.
- Any exercise is better than no exercise.
- Increase (or start) an exercise regimen by gradually incorporating activities that you enjoy into your routine.
- Exercise is an important component of long-term weight management—and once you lose the weight you want to, you won't want to gain it back!

STAY
SMART

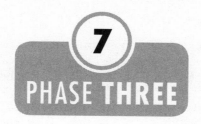

PHASE **THREE**
7

Eat Smarter

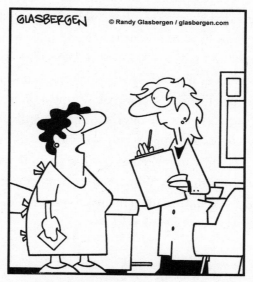

"Which 'sensible diet' do you want me
to follow? I found 123,942 of them
on the Internet!"

The food you eat can either be the safest and most
powerful form of medicine or the slowest form of
poison.

Amy Wigmore, holistic health practitioner

You've come such a long way—congratulate yourself! You now understand what it took me more than twenty years of my life to figure out: there are no magic, quick-fix diets that will work for long-term weight loss. However, eating for your health (and weight loss) is actually a lot easier then constantly dieting! The first time I ever sat down with a nutritionist, I was sixteen years old. After years as a dancer and plenty of personal dieting disasters, I was in desperate need of nutritional advice. She began to explain to me some of the science of weight management that can be found in this book. The nutritionists I've done research with since then have only reiterated her main point: eating well does not have to be hard, but you have to know what you are doing! Nutritional science, the psychology of eating, and exercise physiology are complex topics, but you don't need to understand all the details; you just need to know the basics. Understanding these basics will help you find your way through all of the confusing information about calories, fat, carbs, sugar, and what does and doesn't lead to weight loss and weight management. This chapter will provide you with additional information about *how* to implement a gradual approach to weight loss and management so you can succeed today, tomorrow, and for the rest of your life!

Deconstructing the Calorie

Let's talk calories—not just how many or how few will help you lose weight, but what a calorie actually is. You probably learned in high school chemistry class that a calorie is a unit of measurement used to describe the energy potential of a substance. More specifically, the calorie from chemistry class is the unit of energy equal to the heat required to raise the temperature of one gram of water one degree Celsius. The nutrition calorie, the one that we eat approximately 2,000 of each day, is actually a kilocalorie, and it can raise a kilogram of water by one degree Celsius. I'll use the nutrition calorie throughout this book and call it the

In this chapter you will learn . . .

- The nutrition basics—enough about calories, fat, carbs, sugar, salt, protein, and fiber to eat well, lose weight, and keep from gaining it back
- The circumstances that influence weight loss and weight management: when you eat, how much you sleep, and even what (plate) you eat on
- How to implement the advice offered in Chapters 3 and 5 by understanding what sorts of foods you should swap out of your regular food routine and what sorts of foods you should add

BECOME SMART

plain old calorie, as everyone does. But as far as calories relate to your weight loss and weight management, all you really need to remember is that, when your intake of calories is greater than the calories you expend, you will gain weight. Simply put, if you want to lose weight, you should reduce the amount of calories that you consume and burn more energy by exercising.

It sounds easy enough, and yet calories can be sneaky. If you are interested in losing weight and managing your weight, you need to have a general understanding of the calories that you consume and the calories you burn via exercise in a typical week (remember that food diary from Chapter 3?). Once you have this basic understanding down and you adjust your food and exercise habits, you will have no need to count calories in the future! The amount of calories that you burn per day, excluding physical activity but including when you sleep, is your basal metabolic rate (i.e., your BMR or your "metabolism"; see Chapter 2 for more about metabolism). Most people burn approximately 1,000–2,000 calories a day (usually on the higher end for men and less for women) just engaging in the sorts of behaviors that are required to stay alive: breathing, regulating your body temperature, keeping your heart beating, and digesting food. On top of calories that are burned by your BMR are physical activities calories. In general, a sedentary person (otherwise known as a couch potato) uses the equivalent of about 30 percent of his or her BMR for moving the muscles required for extremely light physical activity (like reaching for the remote). A moderate exerciser (someone who walks and does some fairly regular physical activity) uses the equivalent of about 80 percent of his or her BMR to engage in these activities. When you add together your BMR calories and your physical activity calories and a very small category called the thermic effect of food (TEF), you have calculated your total energy expenditure (TEE). This is the calories you have to consume to exactly match the total calories that you burn each day.

To understand the amount of calories you can consume to maintain your weight, you can calculate your BMR and TEE. There are web-based programs that will do this for you and apps that can provide reasonable estimates (try ChooseMyPlate.gov or http://www.myfitnesspal .com/tools/bmr-calculator[1]). However, keep in mind that these are *estimates*. Also, read the fine print on any energy expenditure calculator. Often these calculations are intended to take into account calories you would burn if you did nothing all day (e.g., sat on the couch, slept, sat at a computer and never got up). Further, if you want to lose weight and one of these calculators suggests that you can consume *more* calories per day than you already are, then chances are the estimate is off and you have a relatively "slow" metabolism—lucky you.

Now, before you set a goal of removing massive amounts of calories from your daily plate remember this from Chapter 5: consistently cutting back just 100 calories a day can lead to a ten-pound weight lost across a year.[2] One hundred calories is less than the amount of calories found in one glass of juice, one bag of chips, or one granola bar. With that said, keep in mind that this works in reverse as well: add 100 calories a day to your diet, and you may be wearing a larger pant size a year from now. Related, research suggests that people tend to eat the same volume (weight) of food on most days. But a food's volume is not perfectly related to a food's calorie content. In other words, there are many foods (especially fruits and vegetables) that are similar in weight but contain fewer calories than snack foods that are not as healthy. If you switch what you typically eat (a bag of Doritos chips) for a food of the same weight but fewer calories (an apple or a bag of popcorn), you're likely to feel just as full and save yourself some calories. A satisfying swap, if you ask me.

You'll notice that my plan does not focus on a set amount of calories that you should or should not regularly consume. Although understanding what calories are all about and getting in the habit of making good food choices is important, "counting calories" across your day is not a necessary part of losing weight and weight management. Rather than asking you to do a mathematical calculation every time you sit down to eat, my recommendation goes like this: if you want to lose weight, eat less than you currently do. Of course, you have to know how you currently eat to know how to eat better. Once you've followed my advice from Chapters 3 and 5, you will be well on your way to reducing your caloric intake by *at least* 100 calories a day (just by swapping out some of your drink and snack choices). By doing this you will gradually reduce your calorie consumption, and you don't have to add up your caloric intake over the course of the day. As you figure out drinks, snacks, desserts, and meals that you know are of a reasonable calorie content and that you like, stick to a healthy repertoire of these foods and beverages on most days. Getting in some food habits—for example breakfasts you usually have and snacks you keep on hand—will make grocery shopping a lot easier and will eliminate the need to keep checking on the nutritional values of everything you put into your mouth. Keeping track of every calorie that you consume is not a great long-term approach to weight management. Eating should be fun; it should not feel like math homework.

An Interview with a Registered Dietician

In the process of writing this book, I conferred with my colleagues from the department of nutritional sciences at Rutgers University (in particular, Dr. Joseph Dixon and Peggy Policastro). While I was writing this book, Peggy agreed to let me interview her about some of the issues in nutrition that can be confusing to people. Peggy is a registered dietician, teaches classes in nutrition, and conducts research at Rutgers. She also puts her expertise to work consulting with dining services on campus.

CM: If people are interested in "watching" or "counting" a particular kind of value—carbs, calories, sugar, fat—to try to lose weight, what do you recommend they focus on and why?

PP: All foods have a place in our diet—in moderation. Even fat has a place in our diet—it makes us feel full for a long period of time. If we try to exclude a particular nutrient, we tend to miss it and ultimately return to eating (and often overeating) it. However, the most successful long-term approach to weight loss is to lower caloric intake.

CM: Is a calorie just a calorie? Are some calories (e.g., from fat) worse for us than others?

PP: Yes; a calorie is a calorie. Some calories are demonized, but our bodies handle all calories the same way. They're all broken into glucose or free fatty acids to "feed" our brain and muscles. A calorie from fat is not really different (in terms of weight regulation) than is a calorie from carbohydrates. Although some research focuses on the particular ways that our bodies utilize carbohydrates versus fats versus sugars, there is no long-term research to show that calories from one kind of nutrient lead to weight loss or gain differently than from other nutrients. In fact, early nutritionists in the late 1800s and early 1900s confirmed this fact over and over again.

CM: Why have low-carb diets been so popular?

PP: Diets before the Atkins Diet (and other low-carb approaches) asked people to exclude foods like red meat and ice cream from what they ate. Then, the Atkins Diet came along and said that we can eat those things—and still lose weight. This was a welcome excuse for many to eat foods that they may have felt guilty about consuming before. The result was that people started to demonize carbohydrates. When people stop eating carbohydrates, they are likely to initially lose some weight quickly, because carbohydrates retain fluids. Losing a few pounds of water weight quickly is not the same thing as losing a "real" amount of weight long-term. All these sorts of trends come and go, though. There is no magic in any diet. If you want to lose weight, you must eat less (i.e., lower your caloric intake) and exercise more (expend more calories).

CM: What's the big deal with sugar these days? Sugar and artificial sugar (artificial sweeteners) are always being described as bad for you—are they?

PP: The main problem I see with artificial sweeteners is that we know that there are no calories in these sweeteners and this seems to turn off our ability to regulate how many calories we've consumed. We get used to food tasting sweet without calories in it, and then we find ourselves up against regular sugar (which has a lot of calories per ounce) and we don't have the self-regulation we need to have with regular sugar.

Of course, moderation in any food we eat is important. Even zero-calorie artificially sweetened soda should be consumed in moderation. It is not a healthier option than water or low-fat milk. We don't want artificially sweetened foods to replace foods that are better for us nutritionally.

CM: What are your thoughts about some of the diet plans that are currently popular?

PP: If your overall caloric intake goes down, then you are going to lose weight. It is not a good idea to fast, although some current plans prescribe this. It is normal to eat more on some days than others, but skipping meals or severely restricting caloric intake is going to leave you feeling sluggish and tired. It is impossible to be physically active without eating. It's like trying to run a car without any gas in it.

Overall, the rules I suggest are to eat breakfast every day, eat five servings of fruits and veggies each day, try to exercise each day, and limit television and screen time. That doesn't make for an exciting "diet plan," but it will effectively help people to manage their weight.

CM: Do you have any final "words of wisdom" for people trying to lose weight and keep it off?

PP: What I recommend to people to help them to lose weight is not always sexy, but it is what works. Weight-loss books change; most of them don't stick around because they don't work. To be healthy and lose weight, you have to change your habits. You also have to understand why you are eating. Convenience, habits, and our emotions are all an important part of our food choices. If we all stopped eating when we were full and followed some basic nutritional guidelines, we wouldn't be in the midst of an obesity epidemic.

Fat Facts

During the 1990s, low-fat and nonfat foods became very popular. Products ranging from salad dressings to bread were packaged with labels indicating that they were "fat free." This encouraged many people to consume these products with little or no guilt. This also led to what Michael Pollan has referred to as the "Snackwell's Phenomenon."[3] Snackwell's is a brand of cakes, cookies, and other sweet and snack (primarily nonnutritive) foods that have become very popular by capitalizing on this marketing approach. The Snackwell's Phenomenon refers to the fact that people tend to eat more foods when they think they are fat free (or are not a source of guilt for some other reason). However, let's say you eat two Snackwell's cookies (at 150 calories each) because they are fat free. You'd actually be much better off eating one regular cookie, containing fat, at 200 calories—not to mention more satisfied! Fat free and calorie free are not the same thing. Remember, the fat content of foods is not as important for weight loss as the calorie content. Excess calories are what make you gain weight.

So if the fat content of foods isn't as important as calories, why is fat bad for you? Fat is more calorie dense than other food nutrients such as carbohydrates or proteins. Fatty foods are often satisfying, and there is research to indicate that we are "hard wired" to crave fat. Thousands of years ago, it made sense for humans to desire fatty foods because food was scarce. Eating something that was calorie dense and satisfying was logical in a food environment when it wasn't clear when or where your next meal would come from. Fast forward to today's food environment. It is nothing like it was a thousand—or even fifty—years ago. Today, high-fat foods are everywhere: pizza, burgers, French fries, and that whipped cream on your latte. Anything that is processed or fried is likely to have an especially high fat content. And I probably don't have to tell you how easy it is to consume too many calories if you are eating foods high in fat. I mean, who eats just one slice of pizza or one handful of fries? But remember, it isn't the fat itself that will make you gain weight; it is the fact that fat is high in calories that is the main problem.

It is important to understand that there are different kinds of fat and that having some fat in your diet is actually good for you. For example, you may have heard people say that nuts or avocados contain "good fat." These foods contain unsaturated fats that do not have the same effect on your cholesterol and heart health as do saturated fats. In contrast, saturated fats raise your blood cholesterol, and limiting your intake of foods high in saturated fats—meat, whole milk (not low-fat milk), dairy products—can lower your blood cholesterol. Fat intake is also associated with health problems, including heart disease and some cancers.[4]

The bottom line: there is reason to be mindful of the amount of fat that you consume, particularly saturated fats. However, you actually need to consume some fat! Fat in and of itself will not make you gain weight. For example, if you normally eat 2,000 calories each day and 200 come from fat, your weight will not change if you increase this to 400 calories from fat but maintain the total of 2,000 calories. This is why some people can stay very skinny even while eating peanut butter sandwiches regularly; they are high in unsaturated fat, and if caloric intake is kept low, weight can be kept low as well.

Sneaky Sugars and Salt

Pretty much every processed food (food that is not a natural product such as fruits, vegetables, or eggs) contains sugar and salt. I'm not just referring to the sweets you eat or the obviously salty French fries. Check the food labels on your bread, cereal, granola bars, condiments, chicken nuggets, soup, and frozen and canned fruits and vegetables. Sugar and salt are often called by names other than "sugar" and "salt." Salt may be called sodium chloride, and it plays a preservative role in many foods we consume and makes most foods taste better; thus, it is everywhere. A typical slice of bread contains between 100 and 200 milligrams of salt. A number of Weight Watchers TV dinners contain nearly 900 milligrams of salt. The American Heart Association recommends that all of us keep our salt intake to around 2,400 milligrams.[5] That's only one teaspoon of salt! Most people consume 3,400 milligrams daily. So it isn't a bad idea to reduce your salt intake by about 1,000 milligrams a day. In fact, the American Heart Association even advises that high-risk groups (e.g., middle-aged and older adults, African Americans) reduce their salt intake to about 1,500 milligrams. Salt in and of itself will not make us gain weight, but it contributes to water retention and oftentimes constipation. Neither of these things leave us feeling good, and, because of salt's potentially detrimental effects on our overall health, awareness of our salt consumption is warranted.

Sugar may go by names such as high fructose corn syrup, cane sugar, dextrose, fruit juice concentrate, or one of dozens of other names. Similar to salt, sugar makes things taste better. We're all becoming so used to sweet foods that we don't like bread (or soup or chicken nuggets or cereal) without sugar in it. Manufacturers know this and load up food products with salt and sugar to make them appetizing; their goal is not to improve our health but to get us to buy their products. Some recent research even suggests that we start to crave these sugary, salty concoctions and can feel "addicted" to them; the more we are exposed to them, the more we want them.[6]

Sugar has been demonized even more than salt in recent years. Research suggests that our bodies metabolize sugar more rapidly than we metabolize other food products, making the consumption of sugar particularly detrimental.[7] Sugar consumption is linked directly to an increase in diabetes rates in the past decade. Researchers have even asserted that obesity is not the real problem contributing to negative health consequences in recent decades but that our increase in sugar consumption is the culprit.[8] However, the evidence supporting these claims is not yet conclusive; one recent study actually found no link between candy consumption and obesity, blood pressure, and cholesterol levels (phew!).[9] Regardless, adopting eating habits that limit sugar consumption has no downside. Nutritionists suggest that we should get no more than 10 percent of our calories from sugar (about thirteen teaspoons of sugar per day). However, most people consume closer to forty-three teaspoons of sugar per day and six cups of sugar per week. Obviously, we aren't just eating straight out of the sugar jar. But the hidden sugar in processed food products exceeds what most of us realize.

So, should you avoid sugar and salt? The easy answer is "yes, in moderation." Easier said than done! Limiting sugar and salt consumption may be the best we can do. Check the packaged foods you buy, and make a habit of buying the ones with lower levels of salt and sugar. Be especially careful of cereals and other "staples" that can be loaded up with sugar.

But what's the smartest thing to do? Instead of these manufactured foods, eat more natural (unprocessed) foods! Making these changes to your diet will not only help reduce your weight but will improve your health.

To Carb or Not to Carb?

I remember the days when going to the Olive Garden was a real treat because you could get all the bread you could eat as a part of your meal. Although the Olive Garden still offers "endless bread sticks" with your meal, other restaurants have started taking a different approach. On a recent outing I discovered an upscale restaurant in Philadelphia that refuses to serve bread before the meal because it aims to be "a healthy restaurant" (or so the waiter explained to me). Even the French—arguably the world's connoisseurs of bread and pastries—are consuming less bread than ever before.[10] Since when has eating bread become "unhealthy"?

Bread really started to get a bad rap when *Dr. Atkins' Diet Revolution* became a, well, revolution. Dr. Atkins began writing about a low-carbohydrate (a.k.a. low-carb) approach to weight loss and management back in the 1970s, but his ideas became popular in the 1990s and early 2000s. There is hardly a dieter who lived through the "revolution" who did not try a low-carb approach to dieting. This approach is based on the premise that fats and proteins take longer to digest than carbohydrates and are more satisfying to eat. Eliminating carbohydrates means eliminating foods that retain water, typically allowing for a quick initial drop in weight. Skipping carbohydrates, the body's primary source of easily accessible energy, sends the body hunting for a different source of energy. Without a ready supply of carbohydrates, the body will utilize fat stores for energy, resulting in a reduction of fat (and related, weight). Typically, these low-carb diets start with the complete elimination of foods high in carbohydrate value (which includes foods other than breads and grains such as potatoes and some fruit). Then, these foods are worked back into the diet in phases. The logic seems to be eliminate carbs, burn fat, then once fat is reduced add carbs back into the diet. Without getting into the complex biochemistry involved, it is pretty easy to see that this is faulty logic. The body will resume storing fat once a person reintroduces carbohydrates to his or her diet. Thus, the practice of phasing foods out and then phasing them back in will not lead to sustained weight loss. In fact, low-carb approaches to weight loss are unlikely to be much more successful than are other approaches such as low-calorie or Paleo diets, all of which have pretty miserable track records in the long run.[11]

Despite the fact that no-carb and low-carb approaches to dieting are not all that effective, they have remained extremely popular. This isn't too surprising, as a diet that allows bacon and cheeseburgers (without the bun!) has a lot of appeal to dieters sick of sticking to salads and giving up anything that's a little greasy. Further, a simple rule like "don't eat carbs" is easy to remember, and people tend to like direct, simple instructions about weight loss. Plus, with snack foods like chips taken off the menu, the tendency to eat between meals is likely to decrease. I don't know anyone who is apt to sit on the couch and chow down on bacon. Thus, you can see why some people may find initial success when utilizing no-carb and low-carb approaches to weight loss.[12] However, eventually, just about everyone wants a piece of bread, a plate of spaghetti, or a cookie. That urge for carbohydrates can be hard to fight indefinitely; ultimately, people eat what they crave and the diet fails.

The Mayo Clinic recommends that 45–65 percent of the calories we consume come from carbs.[13] Carbs fill you up and are a valuable source of energy. Of course, not all carbs are alike. White bread is usually fairly nutritionally void (unless fortified) and contains processed carbohydrates that are quickly broken down and metabolized as fast as sugar. A doughnut is likely to be high in carbs but also very high in fat. In contrast, whole grains tend to offer greater nutritional benefits, including fiber, which slows down the digestive process, and are likely to make you feel fuller and more satisfied.[14] Smart carbohydrate options include brown rice, oatmeal, and multigrain bread. Many fruits and veggies are also high in complex carbs and nutrients and good additions to your diet, for example, apples, broccoli, pears, spinach, and zucchini. (Although all fruits and veggies are good for you for one reason or another.) In sum: you shouldn't feel guilty for eating carbs. Carbs are not inherently evil; they are a great source of energy for our bodies. However, the rules of moderation and choosing to form good habits still apply.

Protein and Fiber

Most people don't think about how much protein they get in their diet. But the good news is the average protein *requirement* (i.e., what will supply the needs of 97.5% of healthy people) for men is fifty-six grams per day and for women about forty-six grams per day. A regular-sized chicken breast has about thirty grams of protein. So getting what you *need* is not all that tricky to do. However, most nutritionists believe that it is sensible to boost protein intake to up to 20 percent of total calorie intake to help regulate body weight. For most of us, this involves boosting our protein intake by twenty-five grams. Eating foods high in protein is important because of the variety of nutrients available in these foods, ranging from vitamin B to magnesium.

Protein is also important for weight maintenance because foods high in protein make you feel full more quickly than foods that are lower in protein.[15] If you want to avoid overeating, keeping your diet equipped with multiple sources of protein is likely to prove advantageous. Beans and peas are good sources of protein that fall in the favored vegetable group. Soy products, nuts, and seeds are also excellent choices (but beware of the high "good fat" content of nuts and seeds, and don't overdo it). Seafood is recommended as a weekly selection, and salmon gets top nutritional reviews.[16] Of course, there are the standard selections: meat, poultry, and eggs. Below are some smart protein choices that can help with healthy weight management.

SMART PROTEIN CHOICES

Food Item	Protein Content (g)
3 oz chicken breast, broiled	26
4 oz tuna fish (canned in water)	26
3 oz king salmon (kippered; canned)	24
3 oz Atlantic cod (broiled)	19
1 serving nonfat Greek yogurt	17
1/2 cup diced low-fat cheddar cheese	16
Peanut butter & jam sandwich (whole wheat bread)	16
2 eggs	12
1 protein bar	10
8 oz 1 percent milk	8
1/2 cup cooked black beans	8
1/2 cup cooked peas	8

Note: All nutritional values provided in this table are based on best estimates, but specifics may vary depending on brands and exact size of items.

Consuming a diet high in fiber also has health benefits. The Institute of Medicine suggests that women should consume twenty-one to twenty-five grams of fiber a day (closer to twenty-one for those over fifty) and men should consume thirty to thirty-eight grams of fiber a day (closer to thirty for those over fifty).[17] Are you eating that much fiber every day? If your answer is yes, good for you! The health benefits of dietary fiber include normal bowel movements (who doesn't like that?), healthy digestion, healthy blood sugar levels, improved heart health, lowered cholesterol, and a reduced risk of diabetes.[18] And that's not all. Fiber intake also helps with weight loss and management. Fiber is, by definition, food that is not digested or absorbed by the body.

These foods pass through the body relatively intact. They are bulky foods that often take a relatively long time to eat (think about how long it would take you to eat an entire cucumber versus a piece of plain bread), which ultimately leaves you eating fewer calories. Foods high in fiber also tend to make you feel full faster and longer (again, the bulk is the reason).[19] So if you are serious about improving your health and losing weight, you need to add in foods high in fiber, such as apples, artichokes, barley, beans, Brussels sprouts, carrots, citrus fruits, nuts, oats, peas, prunes, raspberries, wheat bran, and whole-wheat flour. Foods with three grams of fiber per serving are typically considered "smart" sources of fiber, while foods with five or more grams of fiber are "excellent" sources of fiber. If you don't consume enough fiber, then use the recommendations in Chapter 5, and gradually alter your diet, one week at a time, to begin to work in more fiber. And, as I often say, go ahead and try to eat too many fruits and veggies! They are nutritionally dense, low in calories, high in fiber, and you really can't overdo it.

SMART FIBER CHOICES

Food Item	Protein Content (g)
1 cup split peas, cooked	16
1 cup black beans, cooked	15
1 cup raspberries	8
1 cup soy beans, cooked	6
1 cup whole wheat spaghetti	6
1 cup Brussels sprouts	6
1 cup broccoli	5.5
1 pear	5
1 whole artichoke, cooked	4.5
1 cup brown rice, cooked	4
1 oz almonds	4
1 orange	3

Note: All nutritional values provided in this table are based on best estimates, but specifics may vary depending on brands and exact size of items.

Breakfast: The Most Important Meal of the Day?

College is a wonderful place to gain knowledge, but it isn't always conducive to healthy eating. When I was in college, I would wake up less than an hour before my first class (even if that class started at 1 p.m.). I'd get dressed and grab "brunch" at the cafeteria. I remember feeling virtuous because sleeping in allowed me to skip a meal without feeling hungry. I'd typically eat just two meals a day and maybe some snacks. I didn't buy the old wives' tale that breakfast was "the most important meal of the day."

It wasn't until I was pregnant with my first child, and I had to eat in the morning to keep the nausea at bay, that I became a regular breakfast eater (one of the very counterintuitive things about morning sickness is that eating tends to make it better, not worse). Now I can't imagine ever going back and skipping breakfast. Of course, I keep a slightly more regular schedule these days (I can't remember the last time I slept in until 8 a.m., much less noon), which makes eating breakfast (and often lunch) before noon not just possible but necessary. I've also learned that I *feel* a lot better and maintain my weight more easily when I eat breakfast, and research suggests I'm not the only one.

For starters, eating breakfast has a positive impact on your ability to pay attention. Children who eat breakfast perform better on exams than children who don't.[20] Although we may not always feel hungry when we skip breakfast, we end up much more distracted than we realize. Not eating breakfast is even associated with our ability to remember things.[21] This makes sense—right? If your stomach is growling, it is difficult to remember the capital of Wisconsin on a test or where you left your keys and what meeting you have to get to next.

In addition to the cognitive benefits of breakfast consumption, there are weight-management benefits to regular breakfast consumption. Simply put, people who eat breakfast maintain a healthier weight than those who skip this meal. This may be because early eating leads to more healthy choices later in the day. The problem seems to be waiting to eat until you are *really* hungry and then making poor choices. If you wake up feeling completely uninterested in food (this is true for some folks), then waiting an hour (or even two) to eat breakfast may make sense. The important thing to remember is do not skip breakfast all together.[22]

Get Your Beauty Sleep

If you are asleep, you can't eat. Well, there are some people who walk and eat in their sleep, but as a general rule sleep is a time when you are not consuming calories.[23] Not a bad reason to get some shut-eye. Perhaps, more importantly, you should get a good night's sleep because our bodies work better when we are well rested. Getting an adequate amount of sleep is necessary for healthy weight management and good health overall.

So, what is an "adequate" amount of sleep? The CDC suggests that adults need seven to nine hours of sleep per night.[24] The problem is that more than 25 percent of adults are not getting enough sleep. What happens when you don't get enough sleep? You become vulnerable to a range of health problems including cardiovascular disease, depression, and even obesity. It may seem odd that not sleeping is related to your weight, but research has found that being tired makes you more likely to eat high-calorie junk foods than you eat when you are well-rested. In particular, the parts of the brain that affect the motivation to eat respond more favorably to fatty and sweet foods when a person is tired. Research even suggests that the frontal cortex—the part of the brain that helps us to be organized, planful, and judicious—is less focused when we are tired. It's a double whammy when we are tired—we crave unhealthy foods that are likely to be immediately satisfying and provide us with energy quickly, *and* we are unlikely to control our desires for these foods.[25] The amazing—and frightening—thing is that this pattern starts to happen after just one day of sleep deprivation.

Fewer Calories for Your Buck

In Morgan Spurlock's successful 2004 documentary, *Supersize Me*, he offered a critique of the fast food industry's (in particular, McDonald's) role in the obesity epidemic. As the title suggests, he focused on the excessive portions of food that we consume in the twenty-first century. For example, the original 1955 McDonald's hamburger was 1.6 ounces of meat. Now, the largest McDonald's burgers weigh in at 8 ounces. French fries used to weigh in at 2.4 ounces, but now large sizes have grown to 7 or more ounces—that can be over fifty French fries![26]

And fast food companies aren't the only culprits. Nearly everything we eat today comes in larger portions than it did even twenty years ago. Bagels are bigger; muffins are bigger; beverages are bigger.[27] And what happens when our portions are bigger? You know the answer to this question: we become bigger! We like these bigger portions because we feel like we are getting more for our money. This is referred to in the industry as "value sizing." Take, for example, the ridiculously expensive soda and popcorn you buy when you go to the movies. At my local theater, the small soda (twelve ounces) costs $4.00. The medium soda looks so much bigger (eighteen ounces) and costs $4.50. The large soda is huge (twenty-four ounces) and costs $5.00. It may make financial sense to order the large—you get twice as much as if you order the small for just $1.00 extra—but ordering larger doesn't make smart health sense. Occasionally, I've ordered a small popcorn at the movies and asked the person helping me to not fill the bag to the top (after all, even the small is a lot for one person to eat). This usually requires me to explain that I will pay the full price; I just don't want to eat all of the popcorn. This typically leads to some of the strangest looks I have ever received. I admit that it doesn't make financial sense to spend $4.50 on a small popcorn and then not even get all of the popcorn. However, if you think of this in terms of weight management, it is worth wasting that dollar of popcorn to avoid overeating. To combat our growing waistlines, we need to start to value our health over getting more calories for our buck.

One reason such large portions are dangerous to our health is because we typically eat all the food placed in front of us. I bet the last time you went to the movies you finished off that "medium" popcorn, and during your recent fast-food trip you ate every salty fry in your order. It is possible to use this tendency for good. It turns out, just like unhealthy French fries, when we have larger portions of healthy food (i.e., fruit and vegetables) available to us, we eat more of these foods as well. Assuming that these options don't come straight out of the deep fryer, we can strategically increase our intake of fruit and veggies just by having more of these foods around us.[28] So it may be worth putting a second type of vegetable on the dinner table or supersizing your salad if you're interested in upping your intake of these foods and decreasing your intake of the less-than-healthy options. I realize this may seem really simple, but that's just it—eating smarter requires that you make some simple shifts in your thinking.

Set a Smart Table

Have you ever gone to a restaurant and ordered a meal only to find yourself shocked when it comes because it looks huge to you? The plate is big and piled with delicious looking food that you are sure you won't be able to finish. And then, somehow, you manage to eat all of it! This is partially due to our growing acceptance of large portion sizes and our tendency to just eat the food placed in front of us (like that bucket of popcorn at the movies). However, it also has a lot to do with how the food is presented. A large plate makes your meal look smaller. A smaller plate makes your meal look bigger. Does this actually impact how much you eat? You better believe it!

Brian Wansink's Food and Brand Lab at Cornell University has done some of the most notable research on environmental factors that influence our consumption behaviors (many of his findings are documented in his book *Mindless Eating*).[29] Wansink and his colleagues have repeatedly found that larger plates lead people to perceive the servings of food on those plates to be smaller and, consequently, they eat more. The color of your plate is also important; the color contrast (or lack of) between food and plate influences eating behaviors. For example, if you have white plates and go to serve yourself some mashed potatoes, you are likely to dish out a bigger portion size than if your plate is red. When the food and plate colors blend together, the serving sizes get bigger. If you want to encourage your consumption of green veggies, a green plate may be a good idea. If you are working to discourage consumption of alfredo pasta, bread, or potatoes, think about setting the table with colored plates. It turns out that even changing your table, tablecloth, or placemat to contrast with your dinnerware can lead to a reduction in overserving by 10 percent![30]

These findings about portion and plate size pertain to both adults and children. When kids are given adult-sized plates, they serve themselves more, and they eat more. If you are trying to get your kids to eat (some kids are picky eaters and the struggle is to ensure they eat enough), give them a big plate. If you want to reduce what your kids eat, keep the kiddie plates handy.[31]

Food is an important part of a balanced diet.

—Fran Lebowitz

Surround Yourself with Smart Food

I understand that sometimes you have so much to do—so much going on in your mind—that it's hard to think clearly about food. On many days you may just not have the time or energy to figure out how to make the smartest food choices. You may have what I call "food decision fatigue": you have so many food choices to make each day and have limited resources to deal with the options available to you.

It may be worth remembering that this is a good problem to have! Having too many food options is a uniquely "first world problem" that millions of people lacking resources would love to experience. However, this reality check is not enough to help you lose weight. You must steer a course through the food carts, coffee shops, vending machines, fast-food drive-throughs, pizza delivery places, and the millions of other food options that are likely to present themselves across a day. You need to change your personal food environment. You have to take charge of your "food world" and habitually make good food choices.

If you want to make good food choices most of the time, then you want to surround yourself with good food options most of the time. Buy foods that you like, you are interested in eating, and are good for you. Be careful; if you only buy healthy foods that you don't really like, you won't eat them and Papa John's will be delivering pizza to your door instead. Probably the best thing you can do to start having a healthy and realistic food environment is to plan. Before you go to the grocery store, make a list. Think ahead to the breakfasts, lunches, and dinners you'll eat for the coming week. List snacks and desserts that you find appetizing and are relatively healthy, and be sure to have them handy. Check your cabinets and pantry before going to the store. Make your lunch for the next day the night before. You'll be more likely to stick to that lunch if you plan ahead (and you'll save time for breakfast in the morning). Some of the foods you might consider keeping in your home are listed below.

In addition to surrounding yourself with good food options, it helps to surround yourself with smart eaters. I'm not suggesting that you dis your friends who don't eat well; that's a bit extreme. But it may be worth befriending some new folks who share your food values and goals for a healthy lifestyle. Being around health-conscious people who enjoy good, healthy food makes it easier to eat well. Want to meet folks who eat well?

10 SMART (AND SATISFYING) FOODS TO KEEP IN YOUR HOUSE AT ALL TIMES

Food Item	Why	How
Almonds	High in fiber and protein An easy, nutritionally dense on-the-go snack that's filling	Opt for prepackaged 100-calorie snacks for portion control
Apples	They don't perish easily	Eat plain as a snack Bake with some cinnamon Dip in some low-fat peanut butter (just keep your PB portion to a spoonful)
Berries (Frozen)	They'll keep for several weeks (or even months!)	Blend into smoothies Sprinkle over low-fat yogurt, ice cream, or sorbet for a snack or dessert
Edamame (Frozen)	They won't perish High in fiber and protein (but relatively low in calories)	They can be microwaved and sprinkled with salt for a snack or side dish
Popcorn	Tasty, salty treat A good alternative to chips that is filling	Can be purchased in portion-control packaging (usually, 100 calorie packaging)
Pretzels	Another good chip alternative Relatively low in calories (fifty-three small Royal Gold pretzel sticks for 110 calories) A good cure for the craving to snack	
String beans (frozen)	Low in calories (more than two cups can still be under 100 calories) Nutritionally dense High in fiber	They can be microwaved or even baked with a bit of olive oil on a cookie sheet (add salt and pepper to taste)
String cheese (low-fat)	Excellent source of calcium Usually under 100 calories per package	Good on-the-go food for the whole family (what kid doesn't like peeling a string cheese?)
Sorbet	Will keep in the freezer for months Relatively low fat and low calorie way to snack, have dessert, or calm a sugar craving	
Yogurt (Greek and/or low-fat varieties)	High in protein (esp. Greek yogurt) and calcium Easily transportable	Typically packaged in approximately 100 calorie servings

Note: These are foods that are good to have on hand when you want to put together a healthy meal or snack. They may not be optimal (e.g., fresh fruit and veggies are usually better than frozen), but having some frozen or easy options may go a long way toward preserving healthy eating.

Try signing up for a cooking class at a local community center or Whole Foods.

Keep in mind that even if your home is full of healthy foods and many of your friends are healthy eaters, you live in a world that contains McDonalds, Starbucks, Baskin Robbins, Dunkin' Donuts, and Domino's Pizza. Not only is it impossible to completely avoid unhealthy foods; this would be an unreasonable goal. But I know all too well how easy it can be to slip into bad habits—a latte here, a pizza night there, some ice cream for dessert. I've dedicated Chapter 8 to a discussion of how to get back on track food-wise after a bad stretch, but it is important to keep things in perspective; one wild Saturday night with too many martinis is not necessarily a bad stretch. It's just real life. Be patient and forgiving with yourself, and revise your previous set of goals as needed so that they will work for you moving forward. There is no such thing as eating perfectly; we are all just works in progress.

- Get to know the nutritional basics of your regular diet and then alter them—gradually—to improve them.
- Lowering your caloric intake is most conducive to weight loss, but making smart choices about salt, sugar, carbs, fiber, and protein are also important.
- Understand the circumstantial factors that influence your ability to eat smart: don't skip breakfast, get your beauty sleep, don't fall prey to supersized portions, and surround yourself with smart food choices.
- Dramatic changes to your diet aren't necessarily needed, but eating less and better is key to weight loss and weight management for the long haul.

STAY
SMART

Restart Smart

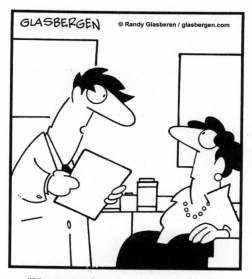

GLASBERGEN   © Randy Glasberen / glasbergen.com

"Many people gain weight during the
holidays. Unfortunately, the calendar
says there are 58 holidays a year."

We all eat and it would be a sad waste of opportunity to eat badly.

Anna Thomas, cookbook author

always "fall off the wagon" in December and on most vacations. In December, I am usually stressed out with end-of-year work and holiday preparations. The weather gets cold and the days get shorter, making exercising outside tricky. In fact, I am writing this chapter in a sugar-induced state of lethargy while I sit on my couch the day after Christmas. The cookies have been made (and generously sampled), big meals have been served, and too much wine has been drunk. I'm tired, unmotivated, and possibly a bit hungover. It is moments like this that I completely understand why people set "get in shape" and "lose weight" as New Year's resolutions year after year. By the time I get to Christmas, I'm tempted to set these goals as well. But I don't.

I've titled this chapter "Restart Smart" for a reason. Overeating is not a matter of *if* but of *when*. We all experience life circumstances that mess with our eating and activity habits. A two-week trip to Italy, the holiday season, or an illness or injury are all enough to throw off your regular eating and activity patterns. Maybe you move to a new city and find yourself eating new foods. Maybe the season changes, and you just can't bring yourself to walk or run outside in the snowy weather. These events are just a part of life and something that we shouldn't make ourselves feel bad about. Can you imagine how you would feel if you accepted that during certain weeks and even months of the year you maintain better habits than during others? What if you didn't vacillate between being "good" and "bad" in terms of your eating and exercise habits and just stayed more "in the middle" most of the time? Wouldn't that feel great? Maybe then you could indulge on vacation, eat enough Italian gelato to feel satisfied, and then resume better habits when you get home without feeling full of guilt.

I want to encourage you to stop wasting energy being upset with yourself when you "mess up" and overeat. You've learned so much and you've come so far—this is not the time to give up! Of course, it's important to acknowledge when you settle into bad habits and have had too many snacks, too many cocktails, or not enough fruit and veggies. Maybe your pants feel snug and your energy level is low. Don't get frus-

In this chapter you will learn . . .

- How to cope with the circumstances that may sideline your efforts to eat well and exercise regularly
- Why New Year's resolutions and "I'll start on Monday" diets fail and what a smart approach to starting (or restarting) your efforts to eat well and exercise is all about
- How stress, depression, and eating behaviors can be linked
- How losing the guilt and restarting smart will make for a healthier, happier you

trated—this happens to all of us at one time or another! It's just time to restart smart. How do you do this? The easy answer is to go back and read Chapters 3 and 5. Assess your weight. Record what you eat for a week. Then, gradually work to improve what you eat. Maybe you feel like you've already done that and you're still struggling. So maybe some more information would prove helpful.

This chapter is designed to help you better understand some of the factors that may lead you to disregard your good eating and exercise habits once they have been established. It will provide you with information that will teach you to deal with these issues and eat smart. Ultimately, this chapter will help you better understand your own motivations for eating and exercising. Once you understand yourself and the inevitable challenges we all face in trying to eat well and exercise, it will be easier for you to establish and maintain healthy eating habits for a lifetime.

People are so worried about what they eat between Christmas and the New Year, but they really should be worried about what they eat between the New Year and Christmas.

—Author unknown

The "I'll Start on Monday" Mantra

The problem: You overate. Now you feel fat, you're disgusted with yourself, and you want a quick fix. You decide to start a strict diet on Monday. Or maybe January 1 is right around the corner, and you decide you will join a gym and exercise every day.

The reality: How many times have you (or someone you know) said, "I'll start on Monday"? Maybe you decided to start a diet or exercise program, but whatever it was I'm confident that you didn't start on Saturday. The weekends are often conceptualized as days to have fun—to splurge and relax after a week of work. Mondays are when we get down to business. Monday is when our "real lives" begin. However, Mondays are not necessarily the best days to start a diet. Splurging on the weekend with the promise to yourself to make up for it on Monday (and other weekdays) is likely to result in a net gain of weight, not weight loss. Why? Because while you're waiting for Monday to roll around, you're likely eating everything you want to eat. You're feasting now because you know the famine is coming. What you are really doing is putting on a pound (or two—or more!) in anticipation of your upcoming diet attempt to lose this very same pound! So don't wait—start today. What you eat (and don't eat) should be a regular part of your life as many days of the week and as many weeks of the year as you can muster.

Similarly, year after year, most adults make New Year's resolutions to get in shape and lose weight. The problem is, this is the same resolution people make year after year—indicating that dieting for the New Year rarely lasts a full twelve months.[1] In fact, 25 percent of adults don't even make it longer than one week before giving up on their New Year's resolutions.[2] And if you are anything resembling a regular visitor to your gym, you know that attendance surges in early January only to drop off substantially by February.

In a study that I published with my husband (Patrick Markey, also a psychologist), we tried to quantify these annual trends in dieting behaviors.[3] We did this by assessing the extent to which Americans make online inquiries about dieting (e.g., using Google searches). Not surprisingly, interest in dieting peaks in January and gradually drops off across the rest of the year, surging again the following January. What we were surprised to find is that these inquiries about dieting were related to not only rates of obesity but mortality rates due to diabetes, heart disease, and stroke (diseases all highly influenced by weight status and eating habits). Admittedly, this study does not provide conclusive evidence linking dieting to obesity and negative health consequences. However, it does tell us that the locations where people set New Year's resolutions to diet are the same places where people are most likely to die from diabetes, heart disease, and stroke. This hardly suggests that setting a New Year's resolution to diet is a health-promoting behavior!

The solution: If New Year's resolutions and "I'll start on Monday" doesn't work—what does? Should we even bother trying to lose weight and get in shape? The answer, of course, is yes!

The reason people fail to change their eating and exercise behaviors is because their approach is wrong, not because it is impossible to change these behaviors. Part of being successful at losing weight and keeping it off is no longer thinking about "good days" and "bad days" or "healthy days" and "splurge days" or Saturdays and Mondays. Healthy weight management means thinking about doing your best to be healthy every day and when you do splurge, not waiting until Monday or January 1 to try to do better. When you slip into habits you are not happy with or that are conducive to weight gain, then re-establish healthy habits as soon as you can, be that Sunday afternoon, Wednesday night or March 1.

And how do you do that? Solicit help from a friend or family member. Remember, it is easier to change our habits if we don't have to make these changes alone.[4] Make a public proclamation about what you are going to do to improve your approach to weight management. You don't necessarily need to tell all of your Facebook friends that you plan to start eating Fiber One for breakfast instead of Froot Loops, but you can tell your partner, colleague, or a trusted friend. Telling other people that you plan to make a health change (and asking them for support) is a proven way to increase the odds that you will actually make that change.[5]

Just because you're skinny doesn't mean you're going to be happy. You can be absolutely miserable when you're thin.

—Abby Ellin, from "Fat and Thin Find Common Ground," the *New York Times*

Mood and Food

The problem: When I'm tired I want to eat. When I'm sad I want to eat. When I'm happy I want to eat. The only times I don't really want to eat are when I'm sick, exercising, or asleep. For most of us, our moods impact our food consumption. To a certain extent, this is okay. If you're excited about a promotion at work, you should go out for a celebratory dinner. If you had a really crummy day, an extra scoop of Ben & Jerry's might not be so bad. The problem is when your emotions get the better of you more often than not and your eating habits suffer as a result. You may not be able to completely control how your mood and food consumption are related, but developing an understanding of this relationship is conducive to long-term weight management.

The reality: Historically, research has examined how negative moods lead to increases in food intake. What you may think of as "comfort foods" or "comfort eating" is often called "emotional eating." Researchers have focused on trying to understand emotional eating not just because people tend to overeat when they are upset (i.e., binge eating) but because they tend to eat foods that are high in calories and fat.[6] For example, people really do eat more chocolate when they are depressed (and this is true for both men and women) than when they are feeling happy.[7] Unfortunately, eating chocolate (or any comfort food) doesn't always provide comfort, especially when the guilt sets in. And yet, when we are upset, we often make poor food choices. People even have a hard time identifying the extent to which food is unhealthy (e.g., high in fat) when they are upset, thus people are inclined to eat more unhealthy foods in response to negative moods.[8] It follows then that emotional eating is, not surprisingly, counterproductive to our weight loss efforts and even places us at risk of obesity.[9]

Although negative emotions are linked to overeating, it turns out that I'm not the only one that likes to eat when I'm happy. In fact, people are just as likely to overeat when they are happy as when they are sad.[10] Although sadness might induce a craving for chocolate, you are more likely to consume *snack foods* like chips and corn nuts when you are happy.[11] It turns out that being happy may lower your inhibitions around a bag of Doritos. However, not all people eat in response to their emotions to the extent that I do. People who are more emotional eaters eat more in response to all of their moods than folks who are not emotional eaters (how'd I luck out?).[12]

The solution: So, how do you know whether you are an emotional eater, and what do you do if you are? The Emotional Eating Scale is a measure that researchers use to try to understand how likely individuals are to overeat when they are experiencing anxiety, anger, frustration, and depression.[13] Take the measure on the next page and follow the instructions for scoring it. Once you've taken the Emotional Eating Scale, then you can actually understand if you are likely to eat when your moods fluctuate.

Please indicate the extent to which the following feelings lead you to feel an urge to eat by checking the appropriate box.

EMOTIONAL EATING SCALE

	No desire to eat 1	A small desire to eat 2	A moderate desire to eat 3	A strong urge to eat 4	An overwhelming urge to eat 5
1) Resentful					
2) Discouraged					
3) Shaky					
4) Worn out					
5) Inadequate					
6) Excited					
7) Rebellious					
8) Blue					
9) Jittery					
10) Sad					
11) Uneasy					
12) Irritated					
13) Jealous					
14) Worried					
15) Frustrated					
16) Lonely					
17) Furious					
18) On edge					
19) Confused					
20) Nervous					
21) Angry					
22) Guilty					
23) Bored					
24) Helpless					
25) Upset					

Scoring: To determine whether you are an emotional eater, add up the points you earned when completing the scale (every "no desire to eat" answer earns you 0 points, every "a small desire to eat" earns you 1 point, every "moderate desire to eat" earns you 2 points, every "strong urge to eat" earns you 3 points, every "an overwhelming urge to eat" earns you 4 points). Total scores can range from 0 to 100 points. There is no clinical cutoff score established by researchers as a clear indicator of emotional eating, but higher scores indicate that you are more likely to be an emotional eater. Research suggests that average scores range from 16 to 25 points, suggesting that a score above 25 points is above average and, thus, indicative of emotional eating.

Source: Schneider, K. L., Panza, E., Appelhans, B. M., Whied, M. C., Oleski, J. L., & Pagoto, S. L. (2012). "The Emotional Eating Scale: Can a self-report measure predict observed emotional eating?" *Appetite, 58*, 563–566. doi: 10.1016/j.appet.2012.01.012

We obviously don't want to deny ourselves the experience of emotions (even the bad ones make sense sometimes), nor do we want to deny ourselves the nutrients that we need. But if you are an emotional eater, there are steps you can take to avoid that chocolate bar each time you start to get a little teary eyed. Remind yourself of your tendency to find comfort in foods, and direct yourself away from food as a source of comfort and toward other sources of comfort: your friends, family, exercise, a good book, a relaxing bath, walking the dog. What, besides food, feels like a treat? When you grab for that candy bar, ask yourself, "Am I really hungry for food? Is there something else I could do right now that would feel satisfying? What else would fill me up?"

Emotional eaters should limit their access to the foods they turn to when they are emotional. In other words, if you don't keep your comfort foods in the house, it is going to be more difficult to eat them when you're emotional (if you care enough to drive to the store to buy a particular food, maybe you really need to be comforted by that food?). There are all sorts of foods that you don't really *need* to stockpile in your home: chips, candy, cookies, ice cream. If you know you can't control yourself around these foods or that a particular mood triggers overconsumption, don't buy them. I'm not suggesting that you should never eat your comfort foods. These foods just need to be reserved for special occasions or when you really *need* them, and then indulge only moderately. Go ahead and go for ice cream with your family on Friday evenings to celebrate the end of the week. Buy your favorite cookies on your way home from work at the end of a long, frustrating day. Just be smart about how much you consume, and try to be mindful of what you're truly craving. Is it cookies or comfort?

Research has taught us that our comfort foods are, in part, learned preferences.[14] From our past experiences, we have learned to think about a tub of ice cream as a treat and a source of comfort. Theoretically, we could come to think of any food as a comfort. For example, women in Western countries tend to appease their need for comfort with chocolate, but, in places where chocolate is less available, women crave other types of sweets. So our comfort foods are dependent on our food environments. We may not be able to change our general food environment (i.e., the culture we live in), but we can change the food environment in our homes, changing our tendency to crave particular foods in response to particular emotions.[15]

Mental Fatigue

The problem: How many decisions do you make in a day? You probably don't think about this often, but each day involves a countless number of mundane choices—everything from picking out what you are going to wear in the morning to figuring out which route to take when you drive home. You also face numerous challenging decisions during the course of a regular day—how to reprimand a child or the best way to make amends with a colleague who frustrated you. At the end of the day, it is easy to feel mentally exhausted. In spite of this fatigue, we still have to make smart choices about what to eat.

The reality: This is all common sense, but it is also supported by research: keeping a mental record of what you eat, or "counting" what you eat, is exhausting. This is one reason I don't recommend constantly counting calories or counting anything as part of a long-term approach to weight management: food choices shouldn't add to your mental fatigue. Studies have examined the mental energy (often referred to as "bandwidth") available to dieters versus nondieters. Research has consistently found that people who diet are distracted by their diets and have a more difficult time learning new information, they don't problem-solve as well, and they have lower self-control (ironic, huh?). One study even looked at the mental toll of eating a chocolate bar among dieters and nondieters. The nondieters were not particularly distracted by this indulgence, but the dieters were so distracted by eating a bar of chocolate they were unable to think clearly. They had too much else on their mind, such as "why did I eat that?" and "what should I eat later today to make up for eating that?"[16] In other words, focusing energy on keeping track of what you eat reduces your ability to do other, potentially more important, things.

The solution: After a preliminary assessment of what you eat for a week, you do not need to keep track of everything you eat to successfully achieve weight loss. You need to form good *habits* and adopt food routines that you can maintain. Work on your beverage consumption, snacks, sweets, and meals (one thing at a time, as discussed in Chapter 5), and settle on some "go to" foods. Come up with a few breakfast and lunch options that are appealing, healthy, and you can eat regularly. Forming good habits and limiting your options will help you make good choices. You may want more variety for dinner (which tends to be a more social meal), but you can still develop habits that will keep you eating well and keep your weight where you want it to be.

Making a personal "food plan" of certain foods that you routinely eat for different meals is a good way to establish these healthy choices. You can spend less than an hour on the web one time (see recommended web pages in Chapter 3) to figure out some good food options that you can then eat regularly. Try to always have a vegetable, fruit, or both as a main component of your dinner. Avoid getting in the habit of eating too many foods at meals that are nutritionally empty. Keep portion size under control. Don't eat while you stand up or watch television. Develop habits conducive to healthy long-term weight management. And don't let food stress you out, or it will be one more thing adding to the mental fatigue that makes it hard to eat well!

Develop a Taste for Healthy Food

The problem: I've spent enough time teaching preschool and elementary-aged children about healthy eating as part of my community outreach efforts to know that it doesn't take long for children to understand that "bad foods" taste good. Ask any five-year old what his or her favorite food is, and you're likely to hear French fries, ice cream, or candy. Of course, this list of favorite foods probably isn't too different for twenty-five- or forty-five-year-olds! We all may like strawberries, but given a choice between strawberries and candy, candy usually wins, regardless of our age. So, how do you get in the habit of eating well when you simply like unhealthy food more than healthy food?

The reality: Americans eat more potatoes than any other vegetable. The majority of potatoes are consumed as French fries, chips, and snacks.[17] Other foods in Americans' top 5 are cereal, bread, soft drinks, and bottled water. There's nothing wrong with eating cereal and bread, depending largely on what sorts of cereal and bread you select. Americans tend to choose white bread or refined wheat bread that is high in sugar and calories. Further, we all know that cereals with a high sugar content taste better than those with a low sugar content, and consumption patterns suggest that folks like their Cap'n Crunch.[18] Want a side of soda with your cereal? Well, it seems likely that plenty of people opt for Coke instead of milk (not necessarily *on* their cereal), with estimates indicating that Americans drink twice as much soda as they do water or milk.[19]

The solution: There is nothing wrong with liking unhealthy foods and indulging in them sometimes. But, in order to maintain a healthy weight, you're going to have to find some foods that you like that are healthy, relatively low in calories, and nutritionally dense. One way to keep your eating habits healthy and easy is to swap out some of your favorite foods for healthier options (such as those listed on page 174) that you find appealing. It is important that these swaps are appealing, otherwise you'll just resort to your earlier, less healthy habits. For example, at breakfast, instead of eating a regular bagel for breakfast, try to eat two mini bagels. The result will be fewer calories but a sense of eating "more." Or get in the habit of eating a healthy cereal instead of Lucky Charms. At lunch, switch your iceberg lettuce salad for a spinach salad to gain essential nutrients without gaining much in the way of calories. Or try a veggie burger on a whole wheat English muffin instead of a regular sandwich. The bread will be lower in calories and more nutrient dense, and the "meat" will be more filling. Use mustard instead of mayo and ketchup whenever possible for a lower-calorie swap. At dinner, bake your potatoes and chicken instead of frying them. Switch a side of bread for a side of veggies; rolls are filling and often calorically dense but usually don't add much to the meal (nutritionally speaking). Cook with olive oil or a cooking spray instead of butter. Switch your regular ice cream for a sorbet.

I review other sorts of simple alterations that you can make to your diet in Chapter 5. There are even entire books dedicated to helping people make food swaps they can live with. The idea is to just change your habits and stop buying, ordering, and eventually craving some of the unhealthy options. These sorts of small changes may seem overly simple, but they will culminate across time, resulting in sustainable weight loss!

Remember, make only gradual changes to your diet; you want to make your habits as easy to maintain as possible! You don't want to get too elaborate as you alter your diet. You don't need to squeeze your own oranges to make juice; just eat an orange. You don't need to make homemade bread; just buy whole-grain bread. It is okay to rely on frozen fruits or veggies to ensure that you eat enough each day. If you want to change your habits for the long-term, stick to a plan that is simple and create food routines. Simple is sustainable.[20]

Staying Motivated

The problem: You decided to lose some weight and get healthy—great! You worked through the different phases in this book and have been eating better and feeling good. However, recently your motivation to stay on the healthy path has started to decline. This is a problem because,

TEN "SUPER FOODS" THAT ARE FILLING, NUTRITIOUS, AND LOW IN CALORIES

Bananas	Fibrous and full of potassium Easy on-the-go snack (100 cal/med size banana)
Baked potatoes	Opt for regular or sweet potatoes High in potassium (esp., regular) and vitamin A (esp., sweet) Very filling, just be careful not to overdo the toppings (i.e., limit butter, sour cream, and cheese; approx. 150 cal without toppings)
Bean soup	Opt for black beans in particular for a high protein, high fiber, filling lunch or dinner (approx. 120 cal/cup)
Eggs	6 g protein per egg make them one of the most economical sources of protein A hearty breakfast, lunch, or dinner mixed with some veggies to make an omelet (and approx. 70 cal per egg and lower in cholesterol than most other sources of protein)
Greek yogurt	High in protein (15–20 g in 6 oz) Low in fat and calories (approx. 100 cal in 6 oz) High in calcium and potassium and lower in sugar than regular yogurt Often contain probiotics, which can improve digestive health
Oatmeal	Low in saturated fat and sodium High in fiber, phosphorus, and selenium Complex carbohydrate that is filling for relatively low calorie content (approx. 200/cup)
Quinoa	High in protein, fiber and iron Also contains vitamin E, zinc, magnesium, and selenium A gluten-free carbohydrate that will fill you up at approximately 200 cal/cup (cooked). A great replacement for pasta or rice.
Salad	Choose darker greens for greater nutrients (e.g., spinach, romaine) Top with low-cal options like mushrooms, cucumber, and berries Fibrous (and high in volume for the caloric content) Will leave you feeling fuller than many meals will The greens are very low in calories Portion control with dressing is essential (a salad can easily be <200 cal)
Salmon	High in omega-3 fatty acid (shown to protect heart health) Low in calories (200 for 3 oz) and saturated fat High in protein and iron A great replacement for other sources of protein (e.g., meat)
Smoothies	Mix low-fat (or try nonfat, soy, or almond) milk, frozen or fresh berries, add in a bit of nonfat yogurt or sorbet for a sweeter flavor A good source of calcium and vitamin D Berries (depending on type chosen) can be an excellent source of antioxidants and phytonutrients High in fiber Depending on exact ingredients, estimate 200 cal/12 oz

Note: All nutritional values provided in this table are based on best estimates, but specifics may vary depending on brands and exact size of items.

if healthy eating is not a habit yet, our motives and goals influence how dedicated we are to weight management. This is a big concern that must be overcome—your health and well-being depend on it!

The reality: Most people abandon any typical diet within weeks or months. They gain any weight they lost—and often some extra pounds. Establishing good, sustainable habits is difficult for most people. But this book isn't about dieting—it's about living a healthy life and maintaining a healthy weight. It doesn't have to be hard, and you don't have to eat perfectly. You do have to stay just motivated enough to restart smart when necessary.

The solution: If you find yourself becoming less motivated to improve your health or just no longer have enough motivation to actually manage your weight successfully, focus on other goals. Focus on something superficial that *does* motivate you, like the ability to wear that pair of jeans that sits in the back of your closet. We all like to think that we are health conscious and not superficial people. Yet would you eat healthily if it made you fat? Probably not. It's a sad reality that we are often more motivated to change what we eat to improve our appearance than our health.[21] One cool study found that simply explaining some physical benefits of eating fruits and vegetables improves people's consumption of them.[22] Specifically, when people were provided with information indicating that they would look physically better (e.g., their skin) if they consumed fruits and vegetables, they actually ate more of them! Including more fruits and veggies into your diet may be one of the most important elements of healthy weight management. And, as much as I argue for a focus on health and the importance of health (check out Chapter 10), if looking better motivates you to eat more bananas and broccoli, then you shouldn't necessarily feel inclined to abandon this motive.

Another solution to the problem of staying motivated may surprise you. What if you could get money in exchange for sticking to your diet?

Could that prove to be the ultimate incentive? In a study recently conducted by researchers at the Mayo Clinic, they paid people twenty dollars for each month that they achieved a weight loss goal, but these people had to pay twenty dollars for each month that they failed to meet their goal. Turns out that the promise of not only weight loss but cash paid off. When given a financial incentive, individuals are more likely to lose weight than when they have no hope of a payout at the end of the month.[23]

Of course, unless you find a study like this, I'm not sure you should expect a payout for weight loss or healthy weight management. However, maybe you can make a deal with a friend who is also interested in losing weight, and you can pay each other for each month of weight loss and collect money when you don't meet your goals. Perhaps you could pay yourself with a reward of some sort every month that you are successful, whether that be an article of clothing you want, a salon outing, or some sort of fitness equipment. Money can be a powerful motivator and may help you achieve your weight management goals. Besides, when you consider the real costs of obesity and poor health, what's twenty dollars per month? And, think about the billions of dollars spent each year on diet supplements, bars, and "potions" that rarely result in any weight loss at all.[24] You might as well find a way to pay yourself instead of paying for products that are neither FDA approved nor effective (never mind, they tend to cost more!).

Another way of keeping yourself motivated may seem counterintuitive: focus on *not gaining* weight instead of losing weight.[25] When we decide to lose five pounds, ten pounds, twenty pounds, or even more, we may feel motivated to feel better, impress the people around us, or wear a smaller size in clothing. However, we also are likely to feel daunted by the prospect of following a new diet plan and inadvertently set ourselves up for failure. So one approach is to just lower the bar and never mind trying to lose—just don't gain weight. Research suggests that this approach is easier on our psyche and keeps us committed to a longer-term approach to weight management. Given that most people gain weight with age (the infamous "weight creep" of at least a pound per year), this may be an important goal in and of itself.

Refocus: Distracted Eating Becomes Overeating

The problem: Are you losing sight of your weight-loss and weight-management goals? Is it time to refocus? Start with one easy exercise: for an entire day, pay attention to *when* you are eating. More likely, you will find that you are talking, typing, or standing in the kitchen and mindlessly eating. Mindless eating not only leads to poor food choices but overeating (trust me, I just ate three pieces of licorice while typing this paragraph and didn't even realize it until I had finished—the licorice, not the typing).

The reality: Research suggests that we overestimate the amount of food we need to eat to feel full. That popular saying about your brain needing time for your stomach to tell it when it's full is actually supported by scientific evidence. It takes the brain about twenty minutes to receive information from the stomach indicating that it has had enough food. This is why after eating a big meal or Thanksgiving Day dinner it takes a while before you realize that you feel uncomfortably full. While you were eating your third helping of mashed potatoes, you did not feel that full, but once your brain caught up with what was going on, you started to realize that you had overeaten, and it was time to unbutton that top button on your pants.[26]

Eating quickly also places you at risk of indigestion and gastroesophageal reflux disease (a.k.a. "acid reflux" or GERD). No matter how rushed you feel, it is a bad idea to eat your dinner standing up over the sink, at your desk, or in the car. Further, these sorts of unfocused eating behaviors disrupt your body's ability to interpret fullness, which leads to overconsumption (and, ultimately, weight gain). Researchers have even begun to speculate that Americans' preference for combined kitchen, living room, and dining room spaces (i.e., the highly sought after open floor plan) may contribute to overeating and the obesity epidemic. Although there is still no conclusive evidence to support this suggestion, it makes sense that our movement away from designated dining spaces that promote sitting, relaxing, and eating as a separate activity (i.e., not something we do while watching television) is problematic when it comes to weight management.[27]

The solution: Pay attention to what you eat. Eat slowly. Savor. One study of healthy women investigated their feeling of fullness after they ate quickly and after they savored their meals (on separate days). When the women ate quickly, they ate more and reported enjoying their meals less.[28] In another study, weight status was linked to speed of meal consumption. Individuals who ate faster were more likely to weigh more.[29] So the trick is to slow down and not wait until you feel full to stop. You need to enjoy your meals knowing that mealtime is not a race and there will always be another opportunity for a meal or snack later if you are still hungry.

I realize that it may not be possible all of the time, but whenever possible sit down and enjoy your meals. Talk with people while you eat (not with your mouth full—in between bites!). Put your fork down occasionally and try to keep yourself from shoveling the food in until your stomach feels like it is going to explode.[30] Consciously working on enjoying your meals and slowing down a bit will be good for your stomach and your waistline.

Go vegetable heavy. Reverse the psychology of your plate by making meat the side dish and vegetables the main course.

—Bobby Flay

Don't Drive Through

The problem: Your schedule is busy. You are at the mercy of others' schedules. Fast food is just so much easier, whether it be a drive-through, takeout, or throwing something in the microwave. It is easy to feel like life is too busy to plan what we eat. But don't let yourself feel like food is in control—you are in control! Structuring a healthy eating environment is a critical part of healthy weight management.

The reality: The average cost of a drive-through "value" meal is six dollars (compared to three dollars or less for a home-cooked meal for one person[31]), and the average amount of calories in a fast-food meal is double the amount in a similar home-cooked version. So not only does it cost more money to enter a drive-through; it will cost you more calories. Not much of a value is it? I'm not saying you should completely give up convenience or any foods you particularly enjoy—eating on the go (in moderation) is something you probably can't realistically give up. However, always try to cook your meals at home instead of relying on a clown, a burger king, or a girl named Wendy to make your food choices for you. As Michael Pollan has famously said, "Eat food. Not too much. Mostly plants. And cook it yourself." (That last part was added recently in his latest book.)

The solution: You can structure a healthy eating environment by developing good habits and setting some general rules for yourself (and your family). One of the best habits you can get into is to avoid fast-food restaurants altogether and eat at home. By eating at home you avoid many unhealthy options and can have more healthy choices like vegetables. Veggies are often harder to get in the habit of eating than other healthy choices like fruit. So, at the start, don't get too fancy with your vegetable options. Focus on buying veggies that you like and that are easy to eat. Maybe "baby carrots," prepackaged salads, or even frozen veggies. Research suggests that the high water and fiber content of vege-tables will make you feel fuller and reduce the amount of calories you actually consume, thus promoting weight loss.[32] As I mentioned in Chapter 5, you really can't eat too many fruits or veggies, but I challenge you to try!

What other rules can you establish for yourself? Think about the food swaps you've started to make. Is there room for additional improve-ment—especially when it comes to fast food? There are probably some unhealthy items that you still eat (or drink) that you don't even like that much. Swap them or stop buying them. If your roommate, significant other, or kids really like those foods, make a deal with them about a re-placement food item that you'll purchase instead. Again, the idea is not to deprive yourself of foods you enjoy but to establish good habits and just keep working toward gradual improvement!

This is also another good time to remind yourself that you should eat only when you are actually hungry. I understand that it is sometimes hard to keep driving by In-N-Out Burger after you see their advertise-ment for French fries and hamburgers. But before you drive through and order that large fry ask yourself, "Am I craving comfort, or am I really hungry?" Sometimes, I realize that I don't even like what I'm eating, but I just keep eating it because I'm tired and I'm too lazy to make some-thing that is better for me. However, I really do feel better when I have healthy meals and snack foods on hand. Lately, I've been stocking up on plain Greek yogurt. My daughter and I both like it for meals, snacks, and even dessert. My new, latest food rule: have a yogurt then see if you are still hungry.

Be Smart and Fight the Fads

The problem: Everywhere you look you will see ads, images, products, and plans that promote dieting. You may still want to lose some more weight (who doesn't?), so these ads, images, products, and plans are going to be compelling. Even as someone who knows better and who has studied eating behaviors and body image for her entire adult life, I often find myself looking twice at a new pill or potion that promises assistance with weight loss. After all, it *would* be so much easier if all we had to do was take a pill and then we'd look like a supermodel without worrying about what we eat.

The reality: As you now know, diets don't work. Maybe they work for a few weeks or a few months, but then you will soon be back to where you started before your diet, plus a few pounds.[33] If you want to be cranky, depressed, and hungry, then go on a diet. If you want to be healthy, maintain weight loss permanently, and be happy, then you need to focus on moderation, gradual changes to improve your habits, and a bit of diligence and persistence.[34]

FIGHT THE FADS MANTRAS

Think long-term.

Protecting your health is the most important thing you can do for yourself.

Food is physical—and psychological—nourishment.

Slow and steady wins the race.

Food is fun.

Moderation is important—most of the time.

Select diet and activity behaviors that you can imagine doing for the rest of your life.

The solution: The solution to fighting the diet fads is apparent throughout the pages of this book. You understand this intellectually, but weight management is an emotional issue for most of us. So you will need to talk yourself off the edge every now and then. Don't jump into a new diet that will only bring distress and more pounds. Remember that you are smart; you are capable of making smart choices. These points may prove helpful to you. Make the ones you like your personal mantras and repeat them to yourself as you resist the urge to click on that internet ad for whatever diet fad will inevitably appear each January 1.

- In this chapter, you learned about circumstances that may make it difficult for you to eat well and exercise regularly. Most important, you understand what to do when this happens!
- You now know that it is normal to fall off the wagon some of the time, but it is best not to wait until Monday to get back on it.
- You've come to understand that your moods may affect what you eat, and you've learned tricks for avoiding emotional eating.
- You've learned how to stay motivated for the long haul and restart smart when necessary.

STAY
SMART

Share Your Success and Encourage Others

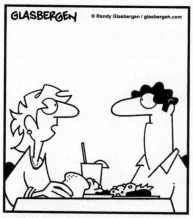

GLASBERGEN © Randy Glasbergen / glasbergen.com

"I joined a weight-loss support group. We meet once a week and talk each other out of dieting."

We can make a commitment to promote vegetables and fruits and whole grains on every part of every menu. We can make portion sizes smaller and emphasize quality over quantity. And we can help create a culture—imagine this—where our kids ask for healthy options instead of resisting them.

Michelle Obama

At the conclusion of my Psychology of Eating class, I tell my students, "You can't unlearn this; you are a changed person now." I ask them what they plan to do with all of the information we've discussed. Typically they respond that that they will not buy or eat fast food. They will always remember the risks associated with what they eat and being overweight. They will have more realistic expectations for their own and others' bodies. But, perhaps most importantly, *they will not diet.*

I'm always gratified to hear these comments from my students, but I can't help but try to push them toward something more. At the risk of sounding evangelical, I want them to "spread the news" about the psychology of eating and healthy weight management. They need to tell their parents what they've learned. Someday, they need to tell their children. I want them to advocate for themselves and others to promote a healthier weight-management environment—a world that makes it easier to not diet, to exercise regularly, and to stay healthy.

I hope, as you are getting near the end of this book, that you are willing to think about how you can make the people you love healthier. You need to not only celebrate your success but share it with others! You are not the only person invested in weight loss and weight management; most of the people you know are likely interested in losing a few pounds (or more) or maintaining their current weight and improving their health. Furthermore, we are in the midst of a global obesity crisis. We can't diet our way out of this crisis. We all must consider changing our lifestyles and promote healthier lifestyles among others.

Feed Your Children Well

Before I had my children, I was sure that having kids would lead to a greater sense of resolve in implementing healthy nutritional habits in my household. My husband and I were never particularly *unhealthy*. However, in the early years when we were living on below-the-poverty-line

In this chapter you will learn . . .

- How to form partnerships with the people you care about—and who can care for you—to develop healthy weight-management strategies
- How to help your children and significant others improve their eating habits
- Your doctor's role in helping you and your loved ones maintain a healthy weight

graduate student incomes, it was hard to always purchase, plan, and prepare the foods required for healthy meals. I knew that once we had kids (and an income) we would all eat healthier. Of course, as most parents will admit, what you think you will do before you have children and what you actually do once you have them rarely resemble one another. Parenting is a supremely humbling activity. I learned very quickly that what my research about parenting and eating taught me did not always translate easily into real life. This real-life experience has given me a good sense of how difficult it can be to feed our children well (it turns out you can't force toddlers to eat the healthy foods you would like them to eat). And, yet, to conquer staggering obesity rates, it is arguably critical that we focus on the next generation.

We must feed our children well and teach them to be healthy eaters so that they can avoid the perils of both obesity and dieting. Fortunately, there is a growing body of informative research on this topic, a great deal of which presents counterintuitive information. One of the greatest and most easily implemented lessons to make our kids healthier is to help them focus on their internal biological cues for hunger and satiety.[1] In other words, don't make kids eat if they are not hungry and don't make them stop if they are still hungry. Children should learn to listen to their bodies and understand what it means to be hungry and full. If all of us ate only when we were hungry and stopped when we were full, there would be no obesity crisis. However, sometime before kindergarten, children often lose the ability to clearly detect when they are hungry and full because the environment shapes their eating behaviors.[2] Parents, teachers, and the time of day begin to determine mealtimes, and internal cues indicating hunger and satiety are given less and less attention with age. However, unless our children are truly at risk of starving, we should give them some autonomy in determining *how much* they eat and when they eat.

Many of us grew up in households with parents who routinely instructed us to "clean our plate" at dinner before dessert was a permissible option. Guess what? Multiple studies suggest that this is an ineffective strategy! Requiring children to eat undesirable foods (e.g., broccoli) so that they can eat desirable foods (e.g., ice cream) quickly teaches children that they should not like or want broccoli but should prize ice cream.[3] Instead, kids should be told that they don't have to eat everything that is available at dinner, but they should be encouraged (not forced) to eat healthy options such as fruits and vegetables. If dinner consists of mostly fruit and vegetables, then it's very likely that our kids will end up eating fruits and veggies! Of course, we all know that even the most heartfelt encouragement will not necessarily lead to the consumption of Brussels sprouts. However, pushing Brussels sprouts and restricting dessert is likely to make the desired dessert foods that much more desirable (this is true for adults as well, of course).[4] So make sure you always offer good, healthy options in abundance, offer fun, palatable foods in moderation, and work to create an eating environment that is conducive to generally healthy nutritional patterns. People are often surprised that I don't force my children to eat particular foods and my kids often end up making food choices that I don't necessarily agree with. But, in following what science has to say about this topic, I know that I stand a better chance of helping my children adopt healthy eating habits in the long run if I don't push them too much. I can't keep them from preferring French fries over green beans, but I can keep serving green beans and encouraging them to sample them.

Parents can also help create a healthy eating environment by modeling healthy eating habits and providing primarily healthy food options to their children. Children will inevitably be exposed to French fries, soda, chips, candy, and ice cream. However, this does not mean that you need to make these foods a regular part of their diet. Don't make them "forbidden fruit," per se, but don't supply them readily, either. Psychologists refer to this as "covert restriction."[5] In other words, keep most junk food out of the house so it doesn't become a part of your children's regular eating habits. When I educate parents and children about healthy eating, I refer to these "junky foods" as "sometimes foods"; it is okay to have them sometimes. In contrast, healthy foods (e.g., fruits and veggies) are "everyday foods" because we should eat them every day. Our bodies are like cars in that cars need gas to work; our bodies need everyday foods to work, and, although they may be delicious, "sometimes foods" don't fill up the tank.

It's also important that parents model a healthy approach to weight management. If parents push healthy eating and then pursue a fad diet such as the Atkins Diet themselves, they're sending a mixed message. Doing so will teach children not only to fear certain types of food but potentially to obsess about calories and focus on weight instead of health. And, because these fad diets inevitability fail, it will teach children that it is normal to cycle through approaches to weight management. However, being passive about healthy eating is also problematic for establishing healthy eating habits in children. If moms complain about being fat, dads reminisce about the days when they were in better shape, and then they eat fast food and spend too much time watching *Dancing with the Stars* (watching others being physically active is not the same thing as exercising yourself), kids are unlikely to "do as they say and not as they do." We need to model healthy eating behaviors and take part in the process of educating our children if we want our kids to eat well and have healthy, long lives.

In spite of all I know and what I do for a living, my son claims to "not really like any vegetables." So, how does research advise me to handle this situation? Offer vegetables repeatedly, prompt tasting of these foods, model eating of these foods, and recognize that actual liking of these foods is a gradual process. Many foods and drinks are not immediately enjoyed.[6] (Think of coffee and beer, two standby options for many adults that are often extremely distasteful on the first try.) Most foods are actually an acquired taste, with research suggesting that eight to ten exposures (i.e., different tasting opportunities) may be necessary before food (and drinks) are really liked. Forcing kids to eat certain foods is not going to be effective and in the long run can backfire entirely.[7] Our eating habits— and our children's—should be conceptualized as a work in progress. Keep serving the good stuff, offer it in different dishes, and let your kids watch you enjoy it. Sometimes, the best goal is just minor, gradual improvements and avoiding the terrible extremes (e.g., fast food all the time).

No matter what you do as a parent, the deck is stacked against you when it comes to getting children to eat well. Although there has been a growing movement toward educating children about healthy eating and physical fitness (thanks in part to Michelle Obama's Let's Move campaign), explaining that eating well now matters so that you don't get diabetes or cancer in twenty years is a hard sell to a five-year-old.[8] Kids live in the moment. And unhealthy foods are marketed to kids all day long. But, there is good news! When kids' food environments improve—that is, what they're served at home, at school, and at grandma's house—their eating habits also improve. For example, legislation implemented to improve school meals has been shown to improve kids' consumption of fruits and vegetables.[9] So although getting our children to eat well is difficult, it is not impossible.

Teachable Moments

The days of the food pyramid that most of us grew up learning about are over. The original model had carbohydrates at its base—which are a good source of energy but vary widely in their nutritional value (i.e., white bread and brown rice are not the same, nutritionally speaking).

As a culture, we've become upset by the tobacco companies advertising to children, but we sit idly by while the food companies do the very same thing. And we could make a claim that the toll taken on the public health by a poor diet rivals that taken by tobacco.

—Kelly Brownell, dean, Duke University Sanford School of Public Policy and professor of public policy, psychology, and neuroscience

Similarly, no distinctions were made among different types of protein, even though lean fish and fatty hamburger are not the same thing. So the food pyramid evolved for about a decade to differentiate between the "good" and "bad" types of carbs, proteins, and fats. It got better but it got unwieldy. It was no longer the sort of thing that could be taught to second-graders. Then, in 2011, enter the Food Plate, a return to a simpler model that presents fruits, vegetables, grains, and protein as the heart of the meal with a side of dairy included.[10] Although not without its critics, the Food Plate is arguably a reasonable, moderate way to teach young people—and even adults—how to eat healthy, balanced meals.[11] Although the majority of Americans do not follow the guideline proposed that "about half of your nutritional intake should be from fruits and vegetables," I think it is a great goal to strive toward. The Food Plate web page (www.ChooseMyPlate.gov) also includes a wealth of information that is both educational and practical.

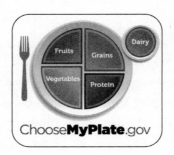

My Food Plate has infiltrated the elementary school curriculum, as evidenced not only by the research I do but by the handouts my own kids bring home from school. This is great, but it still isn't enough. Each year $870 million is spent to market foods and beverages to kids in the United States.[12] These efforts are concentrated almost exclusively on advertising cereal, fast food, and snack foods.[13] The bad news for health is that these ads are extremely effective.[14] One study even indicates that when celebrities endorse food products such as Oreos (Serena Williams), Papa John's pizza (Peyton Manning), or Pepsi (Beyoncé Knowles), kids end up eating more of those foods.[15] Where are the commercials featuring celebrity endorsements of fruits and vegetables? Where would the budget for such endorsements come from? Or, better yet, where are the celebrities willing to volunteer for such a cause? Although there is a certain degree of pressure to improve the health-related messages aimed at children, some companies will always favor money over a sense of responsibility for protecting children's dietary habits.[16]

The news is not all bad, however. Some companies are making moves in the right direction. McDonald's has committed to *not* marketing some of its unhealthier options to children and now includes fruits and vegetables on its menu.[17] Burger King has produced a "healthier" French fry (called "satisfries") that are 30 percent lower in calories and 40 percent lower in fat than its competitor's (McDonald's) fries.[18] Cereals marketed to kids are now lower in sodium and sugar and higher in fiber than they were just a few years ago.[19] However, there is plenty of work to be done; 97 percent of children's meals at the top restaurant chains are still unhealthy.[20]

My eight-year-old was shocked the other day when I tried to explain to him that people who make food don't typically care whether it is healthy for you. They care about selling their product. He had innocently assumed that people were not "allowed" to make cereal, hamburgers, or doughnuts if they were completely nutritionally depleted. He understands that some foods are "everyday foods" while others are "sometimes foods," but it was incomprehensible to him that foods that posed a health risk were allowed to be produced. Of course, what is tricky in thinking about foods as a "risk" is that a single consumption of any food will not instantly kill you. No matter how much chocolate you eat, you are unlikely to actually overdose on it the way you can overdose on heroin. Food does its damage (and provides its benefits) slowly, over time. However, public health messages directed at children with the aim of improving their eating and physical activity patterns seem be having a positive effect by encouraging youths to exercise more, eat more fruits and vegetables, and consume less sugar.[21]

One More Reason to Help Kids Eat Well

Researchers at the University of Bristol in the United Kingdom have recently discovered that the risk of becoming obese later in life may begin earlier in life than we'd assumed and the consequences of obesity may be more diverse and far reaching than those of us in the medical community had imagined.

Dr. Kate Northstone and colleagues have found that children's IQ is linked with the food they consume.[22] Specifically, after studying nearly 4,000 children when they were 3, 4, 5, and 8.5 years of age, her research team found a link between kids' food intake at 3 years and their IQ a little over 5 years later. Kids who ate more processed foods (high in sugar and fat intake) had lower IQs than did kids who ate healthier foods (e.g., fruits and vegetables). The researchers controlled for many factors that may explain the link between diet and intelligence, so it seems that food may really affect not only our developing bodies but also our developing minds early in life. This sort of study is just one more reminder to parents that, even if our kids don't get excited when offered vegetables at dinnertime, it is important to keep offering them and encouraging their consumption. Not only will broccoli contribute to their health; it might even increase their SAT scores!

Gently Encourage Your Loved Ones

In addition to looking out for the health of your children, there is plenty you can do to help your grown-up loved ones become healthier. There is a clear link between the weight of our good friends and partners and our own weight, so helping to keep those around us svelte may indirectly help keep us fit as well.[23] A win-win!

It seems that when we are in a romantic relationship, we tend to compare our weight status to our partner's.[24] If we are heavier than our partner, we have more concerns about our body and weight.[25] When we are overweight and our partner is not, we look at our partner and are reminded of our own overweight status, making us more concerned about our bodies and weight.[26] However, instead of comparing, we should conspire. View your significant other, friend, or family member as a teammate, and work together at healthy weight management.

Of course, a great way to lose friends and upset a partner is to point out the calorie content of the foods they are eating. If you are concerned about a loved one's health because of his or her weight status or a friend or family member has expressed concern to you about his or her weight, then you will need to tread carefully during the ensuing conversation. We are all fairly sensitive and feel some vulnerability when it comes to our appearance, and we take what we eat personally, so engaging in any discussion of eating and weight with people we care about can be risky.

My best advice: don't ever use the "F word" (fat). Instead, focus on health. Telling your boyfriend he is fat is not going to motivate him to lose weight. Most people are aware of their own weight and have some idea as to whether they are overweight.[27] Using the "F word" is only going to be hurtful and embarrassing, and it will lead to anger and resentment. If you really care about what someone weighs, then tell that person that you have concerns about his or her health. Remember too that how you say something is as important as what you say.[28] Be caring, and assess your weight status together following the instructions in

Chapter 3 (weigh yourself, measure your height, compute your BMI—or let an app like SmartenFit do it for you). Just remember, criticizing someone as fat always makes you sound mean and superficial. Talking about health and the importance of taking care of one's body to ensure a long life makes you a nice, helpful, and caring friend and partner.

Keep in mind that your friends and loved ones who are interested in losing weight have probably already tried several approaches to weight loss. And, very likely, these past approaches have been unsuccessful. It is easy for them to feel discouraged. Remember, you've been there, too! What is helpful is encouragement, being told, "You can do it!" Even little bits of supportive advice may go a long way. For example, give your friends a tip, such as telling them about your kids' newfound love for edamame. (A vegetable! And it's high in both protein and fiber.) In contrast, don't ever ask, "Are you really still hungry?" And asking, "Are you sure you should eat that?" is unlikely to do anything but make the receiver of that question defiant. Do these questions seem like the sort of thing we might find ourselves asking our kids and not our adult friends? Believe it or not, in my research I find that people ask these questions of their significant others all the time. Remember, if you want to help your loved ones, always suggest healthy behaviors with inspiration and kindness.

If you are concerned about someone's health, you might even consider making a lifestyle change with him or her. You can tell your significant other that you think you both should begin an exercise regimen. Maybe you could ride your bikes on the weekend or start going for walks after dinner. Making changes to your lifestyle—whether it is picking up an exercise routine or changing the foods you eat for breakfast—is easier and more enjoyable if someone is doing it with you. My husband and I are constantly juggling our schedules to provide each other with time to exercise. We don't actually physically exercise together all that often, but having a partner who encourages you and helps you find the time to exercise makes it a whole lot easier to stay motivated and in shape.

Helping to keep our loved ones and ourselves stay healthy may not always be convenient; it may require extra trips to the grocery store, encouragement, and the purchase of exercise equipment. However, it will allow you to spend many extra years with the people you love.

Of course, everyone should feel a sense of autonomy over their bodies and what they put into their bodies. You want to encourage the people you care about to be informed and capable of taking charge of their eating behaviors, weight, and health. But you do not want to deprive them of their sense of personal self-control. And, you shouldn't ask or expect anyone you care about to do anything that you wouldn't do. Although it can feel easier to just tell your best friend what she should do, it's more effective to show her. For more than a decade, I have lived by my own advice. I understand that weight management is tough for many of us, and I don't judge anyone who is struggling with these issues. I try not to offer unsolicited advice, because I appreciate that the decisions we make about what we eat and how we take care of our bodies are both personal and emotional. But I do desperately want my loved ones to be healthy, and I don't want them to struggle; I want them to follow the advice I present in this book. I exercise regularly and try to eat well at home and when I'm out at restaurants with my family and friends, and if someone I care about is struggling with his or her weight, I do what I can to lead by example. It's the best that we all can do—show people what works.

MONICA'S *Story*

When I first started dating my husband, he was really into biking. I mean *really* into it. He would bike for hours on the weekend and was always signing up for events—things like hundred-mile rides. I hadn't ridden a bike in probably twenty years. I wasn't really sure whether I even could ride a bike anymore! But, before I knew it, I had purchased a fancy bike and all of the requisite gear. It turns out that riding really does just come back to you!

Now we both ride together most weekends and during the week when we can. We go to scenic trails, have coffee breaks in the middle of our rides, and enjoy the time outdoors. It's an added bonus that we are doing something to preserve our health together. And we both like that we're burning calories while we're at it. We aren't getting any younger, and working together to take care of our health and maintain a healthy weight is more important than ever. Viewing this as a team effort makes all the difference.

~**Monica,** AGE SIXTY-TWO, RETIRED

Encourage Smart Relationships with Doctors

If you want to improve your health, your primary care physician is an excellent resource. It also makes sense to encourage your loved ones to work with their doctors in achieving their weight-loss and weight-management goals. Working with a doctor may not only lead to support but to invaluable medical advice. In addition to these benefits, doctors can accurately assess weight status (which you can also do if you follow the guidelines in Chapter 3) and can determine whether your weight seems to be affecting your health by assessing issues like cancer risk, cardiovascular health, blood pressure, and cholesterol levels. If you or your loved ones are worried about particular health concerns and a doctor doesn't prescribe blood work or other tests, then it is reasonable to discuss this and see whether he or she believes that health assessments are warranted, given your (or your loved one's) age, gender, and health history. Doctors will not only offer some advice about weight management and nutrition, but they may be willing to have patients come in for regular appointments for "weight checks." Doctors are also an excellent source of information about other specialists, such as registered dieticians or health psychologists, who can provide additional help.

Keep in mind that most primary care doctors are not psychologists or therapists and may have minimal training in nutritional science.[29] Further, although he or she may not admit it to you, your doctor may feel awkward discussing your weight with you. The thing is, doctors know that there is no "magic pill" (in spite of what some products claim) that will help a patient to lose weight effortlessly. There is no prescription that can be written to cure anyone's weight issue. The emotional, behavioral, and personal aspects of weight management are something you need to take into your own hands.

However, even though your doctor can't offer a pill that will result in weight loss, forging a partnership with him or her is an important step in achieving both weight loss and health goals. Further, we should all advocate for the doctor's role in monitoring patients' weight status. Health-care providers who are trained to discuss the delicate issues surrounding weight with us should be given positive feedback. It should be the norm that doctors ask not only whether we smoke, drink, and do drugs but about what we eat. Doctors can play an important role in monitoring our weight, inspiring us to lose weight to improve our health, and referring us to other specialists to facilitate weight loss.[30] We can all make these conversations with our health-care providers easier by admitting that weight management can be tough, and social support—whether it be from a significant other or a physician—can help.

An Interview with a Pediatrician

Dr. Karen Rendulich is one of the rare physicians who spends a lot of time helping her patients manage their weight. This is especially important because her patients are children and adolescents. Dr. Rendulich has earned degrees from Stanford, Harvard, and the University of Pennsylvania. She is currently a medical specialist for the city of Philadelphia. Her patients are predominantly poor, ethnically diverse, and many of them are overweight or obese. Below I've summarized a conversation I had with Dr. Rendulich in which she describes how her clinic is working to curb obesity rates among her patients—and finding some success.

CM: Have you noticed a change in overweight and obesity rates in the years that you have been practicing?

KR: Just before I began working as a pediatrician with the Philadelphia Department of Health, the city began developing programs to help children maintain healthy weights. This was fairly cutting edge fourteen years ago, when the rate of obesity among my patients was very high but recognition of this health problem was relatively low. I've witnessed some modest decreases in obesity rates since then, but, more importantly, I've seen a huge change in awareness about obesity and related health consequences. Parents are much more willing to hear that their child is overweight than they used to be; they are starting to really get that weight is an important health issue.

CM: As a pediatrician, how do you talk with your patients (or their parents) about food and weight issues?

KR: All of my well-child appointments (i.e., annual checkups) start with charting a child's height and weight. I'm able to show parents (and children, if they are old enough) where a healthy weight is on a chart and where their child's weight is. I try to explain the child's weight trajectory if the child appears to be at risk of becoming overweight or obese. I don't typically explicitly say that a child is overweight. I talk about weight in the context of a child's family and medical history. I explain that we don't care about weight because we want all children to look alike but because of the health risks, such as heart disease and diabetes. For example, if the mom is diabetic, I explain that the child is at risk of developing diabetes as well if the child doesn't maintain healthy eating and exercise habits. We never prescribe a "diet" for a child. We explain that lifestyle change is important and that changing health habits (and weight) takes time. We prescribe one change at a time, based on the goals that the children are interested in setting. We also have a nutritionist in the clinic who can meet with the children and families.

CM: So many adults struggle with weight management, how do you convince kids and their parents to invest time and energy into managing their weight?

KR: I try to ask kids to think about what they would be able to do if they had less weight on their bodies. They typically recognize that they could run faster, have more fun in their gym classes, and even look better. I try to help them identify health reasons for weight loss and goals. I never explicitly tell a child that he or she should go on a diet. In fact, oftentimes, one of the goals we set is just to have kids not gain any more weight between their current doctor's appointment and their next appointment. Kids are fortunate in that they are growing taller all the time. If their weight stays constant and they grow a couple of inches, it is entirely possible for them to grow into a healthy weight. Our nutritionist also does a twenty-four-hour dietary recall on the day of the visit; she asks patients what they ate all day long the previous day (meals, snacks, what they drank, etc.). This diary can often lead to discovery of poor eating habits. For example, children may have breakfast at home and then get the free breakfast at school, or children may eat extra treats or even full meals at after-school programs.

CM: For your patients, what seems to be the primary contributor to overweight and obesity, and how do you try to remedy this?

KR: Often, when children are overweight, their parents are also overweight or obese. The entire family has adopted unhealthy habits. I try to explain some easy changes to make to these habits. Cutting out sugar-sweetened beverages is one of our first goals. We tell parents that reduced- and low-fat milk and water are the only drinks that kids should be regularly offered.

We also draw blood to screen our patients who are overweight and obese and are able to show the physical health consequences of their weight—even at as young as five years of age. We know that making it clear to parents that their young kids are at risk and changing health habits in early childhood, around five, six, and seven years of age is really important. Although the consequences of obesity (e.g., high cholesterol) are reversible through adolescence, the earlier children start to change their bad habits into good ones, the more quickly their health improves. Unfortunately, once bad habits have set in—for example, by the teenage years—it takes much more discipline and focus to reverse them.

We find that many patients and their families need information and support to deal with these issues, and we ask them when they want to come back for another appointment to talk more about these issues with me or with our nutritionist. Sometimes, kids want to come in every few weeks. We encourage patients to follow up with our nutritionist or healthy weight team as often as they need.

CM: What do you believe are doctors' (primary care / pediatricians') roles in education and intervention when it comes to obesity?

KR: I think that doctors can play a central role in obesity reduction. However, most physicians have not historically been trained in nutrition or weight management. Fortunately, doctors have countless opportunities to learn more about healthy weight management because to remain board certified they must participate in ongoing education. Hopefully, continuing education and doctors' efforts to help their patients eat well will continue to contribute to solutions for this critical public health issue.

Eating Smart—For Good

By understanding the research findings from nutritional science, psychology, medicine, sociology, marketing, and public health, you now understand what's involved in eating well and maintaining a healthy weight. You are now equipped with the tools to partner with your children, significant others, friends, and physicians as you undertake this journey. You are aware that healthy weight management is not a quick process that can occur in weeks or months; it is about establishing good habits that work for you over the long haul. Weight management is not hard; you just have to evaluate your current habits and establish some new guidelines for yourself, whether that be eliminating all fast food, cutting out dessert most days, or resisting the lure of sugar-laden drinks.

I decided to write this book because I have a deep-seated belief that these issues are important and often misunderstood. I watch people I care about skip dessert unnecessarily, hide underneath elaborate cover-ups at the pool, and experience despair and dissatisfaction with their bodies and their weight. This is exacerbated by the information about obesity, weight management, body image, and dieting that is all around us. Unfortunately, most of this information is misleading or downright inaccurate. You deserve to know the facts, the information that researchers who study these issues understand. You deserve to play a role in your own health, to choose to make healthy choices (at least most of the time) for yourself and your loved ones. By achieving healthy weight management, you will not only be healthier; you will be happier and live longer.

I've spent an inordinate amount of my life thinking about food. It's caused me distress; it's brought me joy; it's become my career. I've come to believe that food is both more and less important than most people realize. Food is important because it is the basis of our health and well-being. But food isn't so important that it has to be a source of anxiety and distress. An important take-away message from this book is that you should *not* be stressed about food. We all eat badly sometimes! But by eating well most of the time, you can lose weight. You can maintain a healthy weight. You can become living proof of the lessons in this book. You can embody the proverb that smart people don't diet. Remember, this isn't a sprint to the finish line. There is no end point. This is a marathon you will be running for the rest of your life. So—what are you waiting for? This lifelong journey toward healthy weight management occurs one step at a time, one day at a time, and one year at a time. Get your family and loved ones on board and get started today!

- Eating smart should be a collaborative effort among your family, the people you care about, and medical professionals who can help care for you.
- Establishing healthy eating habits for your children today will benefit them for the rest of their lives.
- We should work with our doctors to effectively lose weight and maintain a healthy weight.
- Smart people don't diet! Thinking about your health as a long-term project is critical!

STAY
SMART

The Big Picture

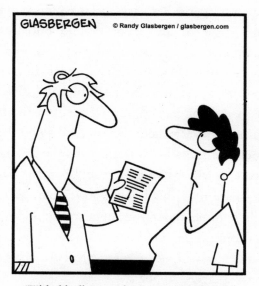

"With this diet, you don't count calories, fat or carbs. You count people who suffer from heart disease, diabetes and high blood pressure."

Obesity happens one pound at a time, so does preventing it.

National Heart, Lung, and Blood Institute

Now, you know how to lose weight, keep it off, and maintain a healthy weight. Whether you want to lose five pounds or fifty, you know what you need to do, and hopefully you're already making good progress toward your *realistic* goals. You might have even started to encourage your family and friends to live healthier lives. But what about the rest of the world?

Obesity is a modern health problem. Back in the "olden days" (as my kids would say), getting enough food for survival was the challenge; trying to avoid food was not something people worried about. Now, most of the modern world has easy access to food, much of which is processed, high in sugar and calories, and nutritionally depleted. Thanks to the wonders of modern technology, it is possible for us to get through an entire day without breaking a sweat. In contrast, past generations had no choice but to make meals by hand. Often, components of those meals had to be picked or fetched from the farm or garden. People walked nearly everywhere they needed to go. Believe it or not, they always took the stairs because there simply was no other option. And people wonder why we've gotten so fat in the past few decades. Hopefully, as you've read this book, you've come to understand that losing weight is not just about your appearance and health but that a better understanding of the food environment—and the consequences of this environment—will aid in your efforts to achieve your weight-loss and weight-management goals.

Our world makes it difficult to eat well and stay active, which is why it's important that you continue to make conscious decisions about eating and exercise. Statistically speaking, we are all at risk for health problems associated with our weight because we all live in an "obesegenic environment" (i.e., an environment that fosters obesity), and, unless we are consistently proactive in taking care of ourselves, we will all put on the pounds. In this chapter, I talk about the "big picture" concerning weight loss and weight management because knowing what is at stake is important—for your sake and the sake of everyone that you care about!

> **In this chapter you will learn . . .**
> - Current overweight and obesity rates and changes in these rates in recent history
> - The dire consequences—for yourself and our society—of the obesity epidemic: deteriorating physical health, diminished psychological health, impaired social relationships, and serious economic costs
> - The potential role of policies and legislation aimed at improving eating and activity patterns for all of us
> - Why a smart approach to weight loss and weight management is critical for your well-being and for *all* of our health and happiness

BECOME SMART

Fat America

In the United States and increasingly around the world, a perfect storm has led to rising obesity rates: we are less physically active, and we have more food available than ever before. Some researchers call these circumstances a "toxic environment." Overweight and obesity occur when energy balance gets out of whack. As you now know, energy balance refers to a balance between the energy put in your body (i.e., food and drinks) and the energy that comes out of your body (i.e., energy exerted in the form of physical activity and even basic biological processes like digestion). If people consume more energy than they exert, they will gain weight over time. Unfortunately, this is exactly what is occurring to the majority of Americans (and people around the world). As a society we are consuming more energy-dense and high-fat foods and being less active because of jobs that involve a lot of sitting, transportation that makes walking unnecessary, and urbanization that has decreased opportunities for both healthy eating and physical activity.[1]

Obesity Trends Among US Adults 1985 Map[2]

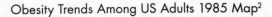

(*BMI ≥30, or ~ 30 lbs. overweight for 5' 4" person)

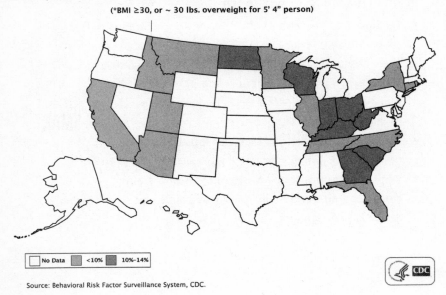

No Data | <10% | 10%-14%

Source: Behavioral Risk Factor Surveillance System, CDC.

Today, 64 percent of adults residing in the United States are estimated to be overweight or obese. As the maps on this and the next page indicate, in some states more than 30 percent of the population is obese. This makes obesity one of the most significant—if not the single most significant—health concern in the United States.[3] Whenever I give a presentation about eating habits, dieting, body image, or obesity risk, I show my audience maps such as these. Each year (starting in 1985, when these data were first compiled), the obesity rates rise. Usually, when I get to the map featuring information from the year 2000, I can hear an audible gasp in the room. Most people can't help but be shocked and amazed at the steady rise in obesity rates since 1985. This obesity crisis is why, in June of 2013, the American Medical Association even declared obesity officially a disease, a move that promises to focus greater attention on obesity research and treatment, as well as greater medical insurance reimbursement for obesity treatment.[4]

Obesity Trends Among US Adults 2010 Map[5]

(*BMI ≥30, or ~ 30 lbs. overweight for 5' 4" person)

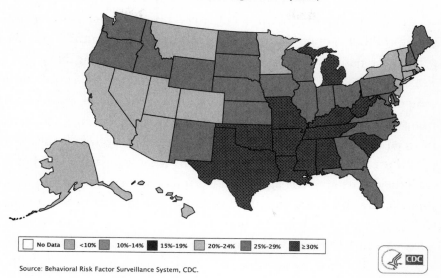

| | No Data | | <10% | | 10%–14% | | 15%–19% | | 20%–24% | | 25%–29% | | ≥30% |

Source: Behavioral Risk Factor Surveillance System, CDC.

It is important to understand that when I talk about obesity I'm not (and the CDC is not[6]) talking about people who are a bit chubby or round. "Obesity" isn't used to describe individuals' attractiveness; it is an important index of health. The numbers reflected in these maps are assessments of people who are at imminent risk for health problems because of their weight.

An Added Threat to Our Youth

It is not only adults in the United States that are increasingly likely to be overweight or obese. This generation of children is projected to be the first not to live as long as their parents did, and obesity is a key factor.[7] Recent estimates indicate that one-third of children and adolescents are overweight or obese.[8] This represents a significant increase in recent years; childhood obesity has more than doubled in the United States in the past thirty years.[9] According to the National Center for Health Statistics, 17 percent of children aged two through eleven years are obese.[10]

These statistics may alarm you—especially if you are a parent of a young child! It is often difficult to get children to eat healthily, and it is typical for parents to worry about their children's eating habits and health in general.[11] Some of my friends find it incredibly funny that I struggle with my own children's eating habits, in spite of my research expertise. They know that my son loves hamburgers and fries and hates broccoli and salad. My daughter dislikes breakfast. Both kids roll their eyes when I ask them whether they had any fruit or vegetables for lunch (and they aren't even teenagers yet!). Fortunately, there are some signs of hope for my children—and yours. The obesity rates among very young kids have started to level off and may even be decreasing in children aged two to five years.[12] Kids appear to be consuming fewer calories than they did a decade ago (for boys, calorie consumption declined by about 7 percent to 2,100 calories a day; for girls, consumption declined 4 percent to 1,755 calories a day).[13] These are all hopeful signs of a healthy trend, and yet scientists caution that these "improvements" are very slight and not enough to eliminate concerns about our children's eating behaviors.

The United States and the Rest of the World

Although the United States is the leader in global obesity rates (with Mexico surpassing us, according to some reports), around the world overweight and obesity are the fifth-leading cause of death.[14] More than 10 percent of the adult population around the world is obese, and obesity rates have almost doubled since 1980.[15] Below is a list of the top 10 countries and the percentage of their population estimated to be obese.[16]

1. United States: 33.8 percent
2. Mexico: 30 percent

   3. New Zealand: 26.5 percent
   4. Chile: 25.1 percent
   5. Australia: 24.6 percent
   6. Canada: 24.2 percent
   7. United Kingdom: 23 percent
   8. Ireland: 23 percent
   9. Luxembourg: 22.1 percent
  10. Finland: 20.6 percent

It is to be expected that obesity may be prevalent in high-income countries. However, this list makes it clear that it is not only high-income countries that are experiencing impressively high obesity rates.[17] But it is not all bad news! A recent report suggests that obesity rates have slowed or stopped rising in a handful of countries including Hungary, Italy, Korea, and Switzerland. In many of these countries, legislation has been passed that taxes fatty and sugary foods, presumably encouraging healthier eating habits and better weight management.[18] Research suggests that the adoption of these sorts of obesity-prevention strategies could save hundreds of thousands of lives each year in some countries.[19]

The Big Health Consequences of Being Overweight

Here are some facts to chew on when you think of reaching for that second serving of pie. Around the world, it is estimated that at least 2.8 million adults die each year as a result of being overweight or obese.[20] In addition, 65 percent of the global population resides in countries where obesity kills more people than malnourishment.

I bet you don't usually think of obesity as a leading cause of cancer. It turns out that current obesity trends will result in an additional 500,000 cases of cancer in the United States by 2020. Obese individuals are at risk of cancers of the esophagus, breast, uterus, colon, rectum, kidneys, pancreas, thyroid, and gallbladder.[21] If we could get everyone (well, everyone who is overweight) to lose just a few pounds, cancer cases among US adults could decrease by 100,000 per year. Interestingly, when obese patients undergo bariatric surgery, their risk of cancer decreases as their weight decreases. This and other data suggest that bariatric surgery is worth considering for the seriously obese (but should be considered only as a last resort).

The most likely health consequences of being overweight or obese are cardiovascular diseases. Obesity is linked with heart failure, the heart's inability to pump enough blood to support the body's needs.[22] In a similar manner, a stroke may result if an area of plaque ruptures and causes a blood clot to form. As individuals' weight status increases, their risk of heart disease also increases because of plaque buildup in their arteries. As plaque builds up in the coronary arteries, blood supply to the heart is limited and a heart attack can occur. It shouldn't be too surprising to learn that the main cause of death in the United States for both men and women is heart disease. In fact, heart disease affects more people in the United States than all forms of cancer combined.[23]

Diabetes is the disease that has increased the most in prevalence as obesity rates have risen. The International Diabetes Foundation has gone as far as to say that "diabetes and obesity are the biggest public health challenge of the 21st century." It even reports that "of the children born in 2000, *one in three will eventually develop diabetes.*"[24] It is important to note that type 1 diabetes (sometimes referred to as juvenile diabetes) is not affected by weight status in the same way as type 2 diabetes (formerly referred to as late onset diabetes, but it is rarely called that now, as younger patients are increasingly diagnosed). Type 2 diabetes is typically a direct result of eating habits and weight status. As obesity rates have risen since the 1980s, the rates of type 2 diabetes have also risen. In fact, between 1989 and 1999 the rate of type 2 diabetes rose 40 percent among Americans. Individuals with type 2 diabetes have bodies that don't use insulin—a hormone that essentially turns digested food into energy—properly. At first, an individual may enter a prediabetic phase, where the body increases insulin production to help the body maintain digestive processes. I've known a number of people personally who, as middle age strikes, find themselves in this prediabetic phase. They have been able to alter their eating habits and start exercising before it is too late. If they hadn't, their bodies would ultimately be unable to create enough insulin, and the administration of insulin (usually through shots) would become part of their daily routine. This typically results in a difficult health regimen, but more importantly it leaves individuals vulnerable to other health issues including cardiovascular disease, stroke, and kidney disease.

When I think of the serious—even deadly—health consequences of overeating (and underexercising) and the growing majority of people who will suffer these consequences, I feel a wide range of emotions: frustrated that people don't take better care of themselves, upset that people don't seem to realize the problems they may be setting themselves up for, mad that medical professionals and politicians aren't doing more to protect vulnerable citizens, sad to think of the human suffering that will ensue, and even amazed that food has become such a big physical and psychological problem for so many people.

I'd have been better off if I weren't fat. I'd also had been better off if the world around me didn't disperse shame upon overweight people—had my grandmother not told me I was "too big," had my classmate remained nonchalant whatever the number on my height-weight card, had my neighbor not insinuated I could singlehandedly topple over a trailer designed for far greater stress than a fourth-grader's frame. The world needs to change in its attitude toward fat people, and that is unquestionable.

—Autumn Whitefield-Madran, writer

The Psychological Consequences of Being Overweight

The overweight and obese are not only at significant physical health risks; they are also at risk for psychological health issues. Being overweight or obese in a society that values skinny over healthy presents an incredible burden. People who are overweight and especially those who are obese are vulnerable to depression, low self-esteem, and body dissatisfaction.

One of my colleagues at Rutgers University, Deborah Carr (and her research team), has examined the link between obesity and emotional well-being in a sample of more than 3,000 Americans.[25] She found that more than 40 percent of very obese individuals experienced depression. Perhaps more alarming, it was the mistreatment by others that seemed to lead the obese to experience depression, not their weight status in and of itself. Being an overweight child who is teased has also been found to contribute to later depression.[26] Similar to the research findings pertaining to depression, people who weigh more seem to be more likely to experience low self-esteem.[27] Again, teasing seems to be a contributing factor, such that individuals who are overweight and also teased about their weight are more likely to feel bad about themselves.[28]

As you'd probably expect, obesity is also related to body dissatisfaction.[29] It is hard to be an overweight or obese person in a world that constantly presents beauty ideals of thinness. In my own research, we find that people who weigh more are not particularly satisfied with their bodies, are most at risk of using maladaptive weight-management behaviors, and may even develop disordered eating.[30] Perhaps most troubling is that individuals who are overweight or obese are often blamed for their weight status, which exacerbates any of the insecurity, body dissatisfaction, depression, or low self-esteem that they may be inclined to experience. This isn't to say that we don't all bear some responsibility in managing our weight (otherwise, what's the point in reading this book?), but blaming people for their health problems is not an effective technique for encouraging them to maintain a healthy weight.[31]

Why Obesity Happens to Smart People

To give you a clear picture of why obesity can happen to even the smartest people, I'll share with you a common eating routine that, if we're not being mindful to avoid, my family can easily fall into. Over the course of a seven-day week, my family may eat dinner out (or get takeout) up to four nights. Recently, on a Monday, my son had a doctor's appointment that backed up to dinnertime, so we went out to Chipotle afterward. On Wednesday, my husband and I had a dinner engagement for work, and we got the kids pizza before the babysitter arrived. On Friday, my son was at a friend's house for dinner, so for a treat we decided to take our daughter out to her favorite Chinese restaurant. On Saturday, my husband and I had dinner plans with friends, so we got pizza for the kids before the babysitter arrived (again!). Although this is not a typical week for us, as any busy family knows, breaks in the routine happen. Because our lives are on the go, preparing healthy food is not always possible, and eating out inevitably involves larger portion sizes and more calories than we tend to ingest at home. What often happens in my household exemplifies the unhealthy eating habits we *all* can find ourselves too easily developing when we fall victim to the demands of our schedule constraints.

According to the National Institute of Health (NIH), our current environment is the main reason people are at risk of obesity.[32] As Americans eat out more and get food portions large enough to feed two or three people, they consume many more calories than they exert. The NIH also cites the low availability of healthy food such as fresh produce and the high cost of such foods as a barrier to eating well. Food advertising also seems to be contributing to obesity, with children in particular likely to be exposed to advertisements for sugary, energy-dense (but often nutritionally depleted) foods. Exposure to these advertisements influences our consumer habits in an unhealthy way, with some researchers suggesting that "for every ten percent increase in food advertisements, the odds of being obese increases by five percent."[33] Finally, there are many barriers to physical activity, including lack of parks, affordable health clubs, and even sidewalks suitable for safe exercise. Long work-days in the United States also make it incredibly hard to be physically active (many people I know deal with this barrier by sacrificing sleep and exercising at 5 or 6 a.m., a choice that I admire but can't bring my-self to emulate more than a few times a week).

Born to Be Overweight?

Of course, the environment is not single-handedly responsible for obe-sity. No one is denying that our genetic makeup is relevant to the weight we maintain.[34] There is a reason so many of us end up similar in height to our parents (i.e., if your mom and dad are both short, you're likely to be a short adult) and weighing approximately the same amount as our same-gender parent. One recent study even suggests that our diet may modify the expression of particular genes that alter our risk of chronic diseases such as heart disease and diabetes.[35] The science of this is com-plex, but suffice it to say that our genes and our environment don't func-tion on their own when influencing our weight.

Our personalities are also associated with our weight status.[36] After examining thousands of people over approximately four years, one group of researchers found that individuals who were conscientious were more likely to maintain a healthy weight. This is not altogether surprising; if you are conscientious, then you are most likely mindful, purposeful, and organized—all qualities that help you to eat well and stay physically active.[37] In contrast, people who are extraverted (i.e., sociable, outgoing) and neurotic (i.e., prone to depression and worry) seem to be vulnerable to weight gain over time. It's probably not difficult to imagine a de-pressed person with a tub of Häagen-Dazs in hand, but why would ex-traversion be linked with weight gain? Most likely this occurs because, although being sociable makes us happy, it also leads us to do some unhealthy things like smoke, drink, and overeat—typically in the company of others.[38] Thus, although our toxic environment bears a big part of the blame in the recent rise in obesity rates, it is clear that many of us possess qualities—whether they be at the genetic or personality level—that may make us vulnerable to weight gain.

All food companies are the same in two respects. . . .
First, they don't care if you eat the food, as long as you
repeatedly buy it. Second, they want to make a profit.
—**Brian Wansink, author of *Mindless Eating***

Why Junk Food Happens to Smart People

I won't even pretend to only like healthy foods. In fact, I love most junk food. If it is fried it is usually awesome, and it can also be difficult for me to resist cookies, candy, and ice cream (although I don't care for any of these things fried). Like I've said all along, I'm not a perfect eater. It's unrealistic to eat healthy all the time! Sugar and fat have a way of making their way onto my plate—guilty as charged. However, I maintain conscientious, healthy eating as a general rule.

It's up to each of us to be mindful and conscientious of our health because companies that create and sell junk and processed food products don't have our health and well-being in mind. If they are selling us food to make money, they will only make a profit if they create food that we like. For us to like that food, it usually needs to contain more sugar, salt, and fat than we need or realize. So, take, for example, McDonald's fruit and maple oatmeal—arguably a "healthy choice" if you choose to have breakfast at McDonald's—and yet it has thirty-two grams of sugar in it. All of this sugar is in this oatmeal only to make you like and buy the product. In fact, this single serving of McDonald's oatmeal contains more sugar than most people should consume in an entire day!

This is part of what makes it so hard for even the smartest eaters to eat healthily: we don't always know what we are eating. We think we are eating a healthy yogurt, but it contains twenty-six grams of sugar (Yoplait original French vanilla; in contrast, Yoplait light vanilla has ten grams). It isn't an accident that we aren't aware that we are making a poor nutritional choice. Food products rely on advertising. Food manufacturers know that marketing a product to make it appear healthy will increase the likelihood of the food item getting purchased, and many well-meaning consumers don't even think (or don't have the time or energy) to do the research to choose a better nutritional option. Even though I know better, I find myself falling for these tricks. We all feel better buying something that we think is healthy, don't we? I catch myself buying products with "healthy" or "natural" on the box or the package, even though I know that food labels are usually misleading and often untrue.

What makes this information harder to swallow (go with the pun) is that chemists, scientists, and marketing researchers create foods designed to not only entice but also to "addict" us. They have studied and learned that consumers don't like foods that taste either too bland or too flavorful, so they create foods that fall in the middle of the sweet and salty spot. They know that sugar and salt is "addictive" (not by any means in the way that cocaine is, but it does lure us back for repeated tasting).[39] They know that foods like cotton candy that "melt in your mouth" make us feel as if we haven't eaten that much, when in truth we may have consumed a far-from-healthy snack (one serving of cotton candy may contain fifty-six grams of sugar!). One former chip company executive was even recently quoted in the *New York Times* as saying, "I feel so sorry for the public," because he knows these products have been created to be nearly irresistible. A fact that has boosted his company's bottom line while expanding our bottoms!

> *If one were trying to ensure high rates of obesity, diabetes or heart disease in a population, one would feed the population large doses of sugary drinks.*
> **—Walter Willett, professor of nutrition and epidemiology at the Harvard School of Public Health**

Soda and Sugar-Sweetened Beverages, Redux

A soda can be a great treat. A diet soda may even be a regular treat. But sodas and other sugar-sweetened beverages are among the greatest causes of our nation's weight-management problem. In some ways, soda consumption is similar to the consumption of tobacco products, alcohol, and drugs.

At first read, you probably think it is crazy to lump soda, tobacco, alcohol, and drugs into anything resembling the same category. I understand why this might seem absurd. But there are reasonable parallels among our approaches to these substances. All are unquestionably unhealthy. Tobacco, alcohol, and drugs are related to numerous negative health outcomes including cancer, stroke, heart disease, and death. Soda consumption is linked with increased rates of high blood pressure, metabolic syndrome, obesity, gout, diabetes, and cardiovascular disease among adults. Children are especially vulnerable, with soda, sports drinks, and fruit juice (aside from 100 percent fruit juice) consumption linked to increases in obesity.[40] Because of the health risks, we prohibit youth consumption of tobacco and alcohol. We know that both can prove deadly over time, so we require ID to purchase these products. I'm not suggesting that we should need to show our IDs to gain access to sodas (although I would enjoy being carded for some reason at this point in my life!), but it might be a good idea to keep sodas away from schools and out of vending machines in locations where youths have unrestricted access to them.[41]

Further, we educate young people about the dangers of smoking, alcohol, and drugs from the time they are in elementary school. These efforts have had positive effects; most notably the rates of smoking have dropped, and it is less and less likely to be viewed as "cool" to smoke.[42] What if kids were educated about food and weight management to the extent they are about addictive substances? What if advertisements for unhealthy foods were restricted the way that ads for liquor are banned from television? Could it become "cool" to eat healthy foods?

Recently, some have suggested that government should tax, regulate, or attempt to decrease adults' (not just children's) access to sugar-sweetened beverages, especially soda. In 2013, in New York City, Mayor Michael Bloomberg unsuccessfully proposed legislation that banned selling super-sized sodas and other sugar-sweetened beverages. The legislation was complex (for example, you could buy more than one soda if it was sixteen ounces or less, coffee drinks that contained milk were exempt because of the nutritional value of milk, etc.) and invited all sorts of ridicule. And yet good scientific evidence suggests that we do not need to consume a twenty-ounce bottle of soda, which contains high fructose corn syrup amounting to sixteen teaspoons of sugar (the American Heart Association's recommendations for sugar intake per day is six to nine teaspoons total). The only question is who should be making the choices—the consumer or those charged with protecting the populace from themselves.

Can the Government Encourage Healthy Weight Management?

Most people want to have public services and amenities widely available to them, such as police officers, fire fighters, libraries, parks, a postal service, and health clinics. And yet we don't like to pay for them—tax time is rarely any fun! Thus, the contentious political debate about health care and the role that the government has in our health has raged on. We want access to good, cheap health care and hope others have similar access, be we don't want the government to tell us what to do. We want our freedom because we view ourselves as rational and capable of making good choices.[43] Thus, some get upset when the government suggests that we should stop smoking, start exercising, or stop drinking so much soda. Mississippi went as far as to pass a law in 2013 barring federal restrictions on what people may eat or drink in the state. Mississippians may have their personal freedom, but they also have one of the highest obesity rates in the nation—and that's unlikely to work out well for them in the long run.

If menu labeling helped 10% of food restaurant patrons reduce their average meal by 100 calories, it could prevent close to 40% of the average annual 6.75 million pound weight gain in the country's population.
—Yale's Rudd Center for Food Policy and Obesity

So, can—or should—the government encourage us to maintain a healthy weight? As with soda, a good analogy for government involvement in eating behaviors is government involvement in smoking behaviors. For many years, smoking was the leading cause of preventable death in the United States.[44] As it became abundantly clear during the 1970s that smoking (and the use of other tobacco products) posed a serious health risk in the United States, public health campaigns gradually began to educate people about the risks associated with smoking.[45] Eventually, legislation followed. Cigarettes are taxed (with some of those funds often going to education about the risks of smoking or education in general), and the price of cigarettes is a serious deterrent, estimated to have significantly reduced smoking behaviors.[46] Laws in many states now make it illegal to smoke in restaurants, bars, hospitals and medical facilities, office buildings, parks, beaches, and many other public spaces.

Gone are the days of airplanes with a smoking section and a nonsmoking section. This legislation has had the net effect of making it harder to maintain a smoking habit—it costs too much and there are too few places left to legally smoke for people to do it as often as they used to.[47] Most important, it has led to a decrease in deaths due to cancer, heart diseases, and other health complications associated with smoking.

In place of smoking as a public health concern, obesity is now the leading cause of preventable death in the United States.[48] Unfortunately, implementing legislation concerning food is complex. Most nutritionists agree that the consumption of "bad" foods irregularly poses no serious health risk and completely restricting ourselves from desirable and pleasurable foods is likely to backfire. So, even if the government "outlawed" candy, that wouldn't do much to help the current obesity epidemic (remember how well prohibition worked in the United States?). But what if candy cost a bit more? Would we buy it less?

As you may be aware, candy has not been a target of legislation, but some legislation has been enacted concerning trans-fat and calorie information. Before Bloomberg tried to outlaw the sale of supersized sodas, he was a leader in enacting legislation pertaining to public health, and dietary issues in particular. In 2007, Bloomberg's legislation banned the use of trans fats at all restaurants. Many people weren't thrilled with this idea, particularly restaurant owners. However, the ban has reduced the trans-fat intake of consumers, most of whom are completely unaware that their food is now devoid of the potentially artery-clogging ingredient. In 2008, it became law that restaurants must post calorie information on their menus. As the New York City government documents remind us, "Just 100 extra calories every day adds up to 10 pounds a year." Two years later, the Affordable Care Act required all restaurant chains, retail food establishments, and chain vending machines to make calorie information available to consumers; however, implementation of the law has proven incredibly complex, and most venues have yet to display this information.

Public health scholars, such as those who comprise Yale's Rudd Center for Food Policy and Obesity, strongly support this sort of legislation, citing evidence for its efficacy and the importance of educating people so that they can make positive health choices. In their words, "It is not about will power, it is about empowerment."[49] This is not to say that knowing that that burrito has 1,200 calories is always going to keep customers from ordering it. But ordering the lower-calorie options even some of the time would benefit customers' health.

Maybe you're thinking, "Aren't there bigger national and international challenges that the US government should prioritize instead of worrying about my burrito?" My emphasis on the potential for legislation to improve health in terms of weight-management behaviors is not meant to undermine other important issues that we need to address as a country and a global community. However, obesity is a serious public health problem that has the potential to impact all of us—directly and indirectly. And I appreciate that there is a philosophical and political objection to be made about the government taking an active role in protecting our health via healthy weight-management strategies. We want to be allowed to make our own mistakes. We don't want to fall down a slippery slope of government oversight that leaves us in a pit of fruit and vegetables because all other foods have become illegal. To be clear, totally restricting all the "fun" or "bad" foods and drinks (however you like to think of them) would not be effective. In fact, complete restriction would likely backfire in the long run. I'm merely suggesting that being encouraged to make good choices is not a bad thing. As David Brooks writes in the *New York Times,* it's not necessarily a bad thing to be "nudged" to make a good choice, and "it's hard to feel that a cafeteria is insulting [my] liberty if it puts the healthy fruit in a prominent place and the unhealthy junk food in some faraway corner."[50] I think the same can be said of making it cost a bit more to buy soda or taking soda out of hospital vending machines. There is no real evidence that the government's oversight of health has ever fallen down a slippery slope into a valley that its citizens were uncomfortable with. After all, how many ex-smokers do you know who wish they hadn't quit?

The Big Cost of Obesity

The CDC note that not only is obesity a health risk but "obesity-related costs place a huge burden on the U.S. economy."[51] Estimates indicate that approximately 13 percent of the gross domestic product is spent on health care in the United States, and obesity is one of the most costly medical conditions. One study of Mayo Clinic employees found that medical costs were $1,850 more per year for an individual who was overweight than for an individual at a healthy weight. For an extremely obese individual, medical costs were $5,530 more per year. In fact, obesity costs more than smoking, with smokers' medical costs being only $1,274 per year more than a nonsmoker.[52]

Even if we are healthy, eat well, and don't need to be told that the double cheeseburger at McDonald's has more calories in it than the regular cheeseburger, other people are not going to make the better choice. Even if you don't care about their health, the cheeseburgers that they consume will affect you financially. Even if *your* medical costs are not high (in part, because your weight is not high), these estimates are relevant to you for the same reason you pay a given rate for car insurance. Your car insurance rate is based on your driving record but also on general market conditions. If you're a driver, your insurer assumes that you (and most of their drivers) won't get in accidents all that often, thus your cost of car insurance stays reasonable. If all of a sudden everyone who drove got in an accident except for you, you would end up paying more for your insurance policy to cover the costs of the other drivers. Obesity is comparable to a higher rate of accidents; as more people are prone to obesity, more health problems will follow, and the expenses will be considerable. The market conditions for health insurance are changing and will keep getting worse as long as obesity remains on the rise. The more neighbors you have who are obese, the more you will ultimately pay for health insurance now and in the future. Legislation to reduce or eliminate the use of trans fats in restaurants, the display of calorie information, or a tax on sugar-sweetened beverages is good not only for your health and others' health; it is also good for your bank account. Scientists know these sorts of measures are likely to improve the success of people's weight-management efforts. In the end, we're all likely to be healthier and have a bit more extra spending money—it's a win-win!

So, Where Does This Leave Us?

Current obesity rates, the varied and serious consequences of obesity, and the projections for the future have led many scientists to suggest that we are in the midst of an obesity "crisis" or "epidemic." Others reject this language as alarmist.[53] However, I have yet to meet a researcher who studies food, dieting, or obesity who does not think that we all need to seriously reconsider our approach to eating and weight management. There is little doubt that our current circumstance is as much a social and economic issue as it is a health issue.[54] Thus, even if you are not currently overweight or obese, it is important to understand that you are at risk. People you love and care about are at risk.

The good news is that many people have started to come together to try to improve the eating and physical activity environments we all live in. Many scientists, doctors, psychologists, politicians, public health experts, and organizations are getting involved. They understand that the stakes are big and the resources are small, but they are gradually making a difference. I've already mentioned Michelle Obama's efforts at earlier points in this book, but she's just one example. The Obesity Action Coalition (www.ObesityAction.org) is a nonprofit organization aiming to empower those affected by obesity by providing education, advocacy, and support. Their efforts include everything from providing resources to parents about how to talk to their children about eating and weight to providing reviews of weight loss plans. Another organization worth knowing about is the Food Trust (www.TheFoodTrust.org), which has been working with communities for more than twenty years to teach nutrition education in schools, to encourage supermarket development in underserved areas, to manage farmers' markets in communities that lack access to affordable produce, and to help improve healthy food offerings in corner stores. One of their mottos is "Everyone deserves access to healthy, affordable food." Who could argue with that?

I hope you will become one of the many people who are getting on board efforts to improve not just their personal eating and activity habits but the habits of others. I'm not suggesting that you need to donate money or even time toward this cause, but there are little things we can all work on. You can implement the lessons from this book and encourage your children and other loved ones to eat well and stay active. You can support policy efforts that improve access to healthy food and limit the availability of unhealthy food. You can be resolved to not fall for the fictitious fads that can only compromise our health and well-being. And, you cannot; you dare not; *you will not diet!*

- This book is for everyone—even if you are not overweight or looking to lose weight.
- We are all at risk of becoming overweight, given the food environment we live in.
- Being educated about food and making smart choices is critical to preserving our health and the health of others we care about.
- We can all play a role in improving the odds for healthy weight management—bit by bit, bite by bite, a thinner tomorrow is possible!

STAY
SMART

ABOUT THE AUTHOR

Charlotte N. Markey, PhD, is a professor of psychology at Rutgers University at Camden. She received her doctorate from the University of California at Riverside in health and developmental psychology, with a focus on eating behaviors and body image. She has been conducting research on eating, dieting, body image, and obesity risk for more than fifteen years. Dr. Markey has published more than fifty book chapters and articles in peer-reviewed journals. She has hundreds of presentations to her name at universities across the United States and at national and international conferences. Each year, she teaches hundreds of students at Rutgers University, including students in her Psychology of Eating course. Dr. Markey has long been involved in community efforts to educate parents and children about healthy eating, body image, and weight management. Dr. Markey collaborates in her research endeavors with her husband, Dr. Patrick Markey, a psychology professor at Villanova University, who changed his entire lifestyle (and gradually lost forty pounds) following her approach to weight management. She lives with her two children and husband in Swarthmore, Pennsylvania, where she enjoys running, swimming, and biking as much as she can. She's hoping to run her first marathon this year.

ACKNOWLEDGMENTS

I will always be grateful for the many people in my life who have made this book possible, especially the students who have inspired me and helped me to think about these issues for many years now. In particular, I want to acknowledge the students who read drafts of this book, assisted with edits and references, and provided me with advice and encouragement, including Susanna Battiston, Gianna Bowler, Jennifer Shukusky, Jessica Schulz, and Julie Wasko.

I am grateful for the many people who have supported, taught, mentored, and provided me with opportunities for professional development, including Howard Friedman, Leann Birch, Daniel Hart, and Mary Bravo.

I am grateful to my agent, Andrea Somberg, for taking a chance with me and for her consistently smart advice.

I am grateful to my editors, Renee Sedliar, Samantha Rose, Amber Morris, and Carrie Watterson, for keeping my writing accessible when I was tempted to resort to the dry and academic and for their many wonderful ideas about how to present this material.

I am grateful to the friends who have been kind enough to ask me about this book and offer me support along the way, especially Lorie Sousa, who is both a great cheerleader and friend. I am indebted to Lorie and Jen van Riet for their collaboration on SmartenFit—the best fitness app around!

I am most grateful to my family for being a source of encouragement and inspiration throughout this process. I appreciate that my children, Charlie and Grace, have accommodated the time and energy I've dedicated to this venture, even though they believe this book to be "probably really boring." I am grateful to my mom for reading drafts, listening to me talk about this project for years, and always offering support. I am most indebted to my husband, Patrick Markey, for telling me to keep writing when I wasn't sure I had anything good left to say, for proofreading and rereading and rereading yet again, and for believing in both me and my ideas.

NOTES

Chapter 1: Just Don't Do It

1. Centers for Disease Control and Prevention. (2014, March 18). Healthy weight—it's not a diet, it's a lifestyle! Retrieved August 22, 2014, from http://www.cdc.gov/healthyweight/?s_cid=cdc_homepage_topmenu_002

2. Polivy, J., & Herman, C. P. (2002). If at first you don't succeed: False hopes of self change. *American Psychologist, 9,* 677–689.

3. Ogden, J. (1992). *Fat chance! The myth of dieting explained.* Routledge: New York.

4. MacLean, L. D., Rhode, B. M., & Nohr, C. W. (2000). Late outcomes of isolated gastric bypass. *Annals of Surgery, 231,* 524–528. Retrieved February 11, 2013, http://www.ncbi.nlm.nih.gov/pmc/articles/PMC1421028/

5. National Association for Weight Loss Surgery. (n.d.). Are you ready to find peace with food, your body, and the scale? Retrieved February 11, 2013, http://www.nawls.com/

6. Hirsh, A. R. (2008, February). *Use of gustatory stimuli to facilitate weight loss.* Poster presented at the Advanced Technologies for Treatments of Diabetes Conference, Prague.

7. Dr. Oliver DiPietro's K-D diet. (2012, November 12). *ABC news.* Retrieved November 10, 2012, http://abcnews.go.com/2020/video/feeding-tube-diet-17469298

8. BluePrintCleanse. (n.d.). Retrieved June 6, 2013, http://blueprintcleanse.com/cleanse.html

9. Newman, J. (2010, October 28). The juice cleanse: A strange and green journey. *The New York Times.* Retrieved June 6, 2013, http://www.nytimes.com/2010/10/28/fashion/28Cleanse.html?pagewanted=all&_r=0

10. Dax, U., Peter, C., & Polivy, J. (2002). Eat, drink and be merry for tomorrow we diet: Effects of anticipated deprivation on food intake in restrained and unrestrained eaters. *Journal of Abnormal Psychology, 111,* 396–401. doi: 10.1037/0021-843X.111.2.396

11. Hanh, T., & Cheung, L. (2010). *Savor: Mindful eating, mindful life* (1st ed.). New York: HarperCollins; Bays, J. (2009). *Mindful eating: A guide to rediscovering a healthy and joyful relationship with food* (1st ed.). Boston: Shambhala.

Chapter 2: Why Diets Don't Work

1. Jenny Craig web page. (n.d.). Retrieved December 5, 2012, http://www.jenny craig.com/clicktocall?s_kwcid=TC-23217-14079912139-e-1714849267&s_kwcid =TC-23217-14079912139-be-1714849267

2. Nutrisystem web page. (n.d.). Retrieved December 5, 2012, http://www.nutri system.com/jsps_hmr/how_it_works/why_it_works.jsp

3. Mike Moreno's 17 day diet plan web page. Retrieved December 5, 2012, http://www.17daydietdirect.com/17daydietdirect/ps/index?keycode=215678

4. Keys, A., Brožek, J., Henschel, A., Mickelsen, O., & Taylor, H. L. (1950). *The biology of human starvation* (2 vols.). Minneapolis: University of Minnesota Press.

5. Stunkard, A. J., & Rush, J. (1974). Dieting and depression reexamined: A critical review of reports of untoward responses during weight reduction for obesity. *Annals of Internal Medicine, 81,* 526–533.

6. Ogden, J. (1992). *Fat Chance! The Myth of Dieting Explained.* Routledge: New York.

7. Wegner, D. M., Schneider, D. J., Carter, S., & White, T. (1987). Paradoxical effects of thought suppression. *Journal of Personality and Social Psychology, 53,* 5–13.

8. Polivy, J., & Herman, C. P. (2002). If at first you don't succeed: False hopes of self change. *American Psychologist, 9,* 677–689.

9. Ibid.

10. McFarlane, T., Polivy, J., & Herman, C. P. (1998). Effects of false weight feedback on mood, self-evaluation, and food intake in restrained and unrestrained eaters. *Journal of Abnormal Psychology, 107,* 312–318.

11. McFarlane, T., Polivy, J., McCabe, R. E. (1999). Help not harm: Psychological foundation for a nondieting approach toward health. *Journal of Social Issues, 55,* 261–276.

12. Polivy & Herman (2002).

13. Ibid.

14. U.S. Weight Loss Market Worth $60.9 Billion. (2011, May 9). PRWeb. Retrieved December 6, 2012, http://www.prweb.com/releases/2011/5/prweb8393658 .htm

15. Polivy, J., & Herman, C. P. (1985). Dieting and bingeing: A causal analysis. *American Psychologist, 40,* 193–201.

16. Polivy, J., & Herman, C. P. (1993). Etiology of binge eating: Psychological mechanisms. In G. T. Wilson (Ed.), *Binge eating: Nature, assessment and treatment* (pp. 173–205). New York: Guilford Press.

17. French, S. A., Jeffery, R. W., Forster, J. L., McGovern, P. G., Kelder, S. J., & Baxter, J. (1994). Predictors of weight change over two years among a population of working adults: The Healthy Worker Project. *International Journal of Obesity,* 18, 145–154.

18. Jakubowicz, D., Froy, O., Wainstein, J., & Boaz, M. (2012). Meal timing and consumption influence ghrelin levels, appetite scores and weight loss maintenance in overweight and obese adults. *Steroids,* 10, 323–331.

19. Ogden (1992).

20. Ibid.

21. The 5:2 fast diet. (n.d.). Retrieved June 27, 2013, http://thefastdiet.co.uk

Chapter 3: Phase One: Honestly Weigh In

1. Centers for Disease Control and Prevention (CDC). (n.d.). *Body mass index: Considerations for practitioners* [PDF]. Retrieved from http://www.cdc.gov/obesity /downloads/BMIforPactitioners.pdf; Bakalar, N. (2012, December 24). BMI can predict health risks. *The New York Times* [blog]. Retrieved from http://well.blogs .nytimes.com/2012/12/24/b-m-i-can-predict-health-risks/

2. CDC. (2013, June 17). Preconception health and healthcare. Retrieved from http://www.cdc.gov/preconception/careforwomen/promotion.html; Flegal, K. M., Graubard, B. I., Williamson, D. F., & Gail, M. H. (2005). Excess deaths associated with overweight, underweight, and obesity. *Journal of the American Medical Association,* 293, 1861–1867. doi: 10.1001/jama.293.15.1861

3. National Health, Lung, and Blood Institute. (n.d.). Assessing your weight and health risk. Retrieved from http://www.nhlbi.nih.gov/health/public/heart/obesity /lose_wt/risk.htm

4. CDC (n.d.); CDC (2013).

5. CDC. (2014, July 11). About BMI for adults. Retrieved from http://www.cdc .gov/healthyweight/assessing/bmi/adult_bmi/

6. CDC. (2011, August 17). Losing weight: What is healthy weight loss? Retrieved July 24, 2014, http://www.cdc.gov/healthyweight/losing_weight/

7. Polivy, J., & Herman, C. P. (2002). If at first you don't succeed: False hopes of self-change. *American Psychologist,* 57, 677–689. doi: 10.1037/0003-066x.57.9.677

8. Polivy, J. (2013, March 3). *Dieting in the face of plenty: Why appetite beats self control.* Paper presented at the meeting of the Eastern Psychological Association: Consuming Psychological Science, New York.

9. Painter, K. (2013, January 30). Survey: Many adults track their health issues. *USA Today.* Retrieved from http://www.usatoday.com/story/news/nation/2013 /01/26/health-tracking-apps-gadgets/1862987/

10. Clover, J. (2013, January 6). CES 2013: HAPIfork is a digital fork that tracks your eating habits. *MacRumors.* Retrieved from http://www.macrumors.com/2013 /01/06/ces-2013-hapifork-is-a-digital-fork-that-tracks-your-eating-habits/

11. Manjood, F. (2012, December 26). An appetite for weight management tools. *The New York Times.* Retrieved from http://www.nytimes.com/2012/12/27/garden/devices-to-monitor-physical-activity-and-food-intake.html?_r=0

12. Klos, L. A., Kessler, V. E., & Molly, M. (2012). To weigh or not to weigh: The relationship between self-weighing behavior and body image among adults. *Body Image, 9,* 551–554. doi: http://dx.doi.og/10.1016/j.bodyim.2012.07.004

13. VanWormer, J. J., French, S. A., Pereira, M. A., & Welsh, E. M. (2008). The impact of regular self-weighing on weight management: A systematic literature review. *International Journal of Behavioral Nutrition and Physical Activity, 5,* 1–10. doi: 10.1186/1479-5868-5-54

Chapter 4: Love Yourself Naked

1. Ogden, J., & Taylor, C. (2000). Body dissatisfaction within couples: Adding the social context to perceptions of self. *Journal of Health Psychology, 5,* 25–32. doi: 10.1177/135910530000500107

2. Jones, D. C. (2009, July 16). Personal communication; Neurmark-Sztainer, D., Story, M., Hannan, P. J., Perry, C. L., & Irving, L. M. (2002). Weight-related concerns and behaviors among overweight and non-overweight adolescents: Implications for preventing weight-related disorders. *Archive of Pediatric and Adolescent Medicine, 156,* 171–178. doi: 10.1001/archpedi.156.2.171; Yanover, T., & Thompson, J. K. (2009). Assessment of body image in children and adolescents. In L. Smolak & J. K. Thompson (Eds.), *Body image, eating disorders and obesity in youth* (2nd ed., pp. 177–192), Washington, DC: American Psychological Association; Ericksen, A. J., Markey, C. N., & Tinslet, B. J. (2003). Familial influences on Mexican-American and Euro-American preadolescent boys' and girls' body dissatisfaction. *Eating Behaviors, 4,* 245–255. http://dx.doi.org/10.1016/S1471-0153(03)00025-4; McCabe, M. P., & Ricciardelli, L. A. (2004). Weight and shape concerns of boys and men. In J. K. Thompson (Ed.), *Handbook of eating disorders and obesity* (pp. 606–634), Washington, DC: American Psychological Association.

3. Davison, K. K., Markey, C. N., & Birch, L. L. (2003). A longitudinal examination of patterns in girls' weight concerns and body dissatisfaction from ages 5 to 9 years old. *International Journal of Eating Disorders, 33,* 320–332. doi: 10.1002/eat.10142

4. Thompson, M. A., & Gray, J. J. (1995). Development and validation of a new body image assessment scale. *Journal of Personality Assessment, 64,* 258–269. doi: 10.1207/s15327752jpa6402_6

5. Markey, C. N., & Markey, P. M. (2005). Relations between body image and dieting behaviors: An examination of gender differences. *Sex Roles, 53,* 519–530. doi: 10.1007/s11199-005-7139-3

6. Palmeira, A. L., Markland, P. N., Silva, M. N., Branco, T. L., Martins, S. C., Minderico, C. S., . . . Teixeria, P. J. (2009). Reciprocal effects among changes in weight, body image, and other psychological factors during behavioral obesity treat-

ment: A mediation analysis. *International Journal of Behavioral Nutrition and Physical Activity, 6,* 6–9. doi: 10.1186/1479-5868-6-9; Killen, J. D., Taylor, C. B., Hayward, C., Wilson, D. M., Haydel, K. F., Hammer, L. D., . . . Kraemer, H. (1994). Pursuit of thinness and onset of eating disorder symptoms in a community sample of adolescent girls: A 3-year prospective analysis. *International Journal of Eating Disorders, 16,* 227–238. doi: 10.1002/1098-108x(199411)16:3<227:AID -EAT2260160303?3.0.CO;2-L

7. Palmeira et al. (2009).

8. Killen et al. (1994).

9. Markey, C. N., Markey, P. M., & Birch, L. L. (2001). Interpersonal predictors of dieting practices among married couples. *Journal of Family Psychology, 15,* 464–475. doi: 10.1037//0893-3200.15.3.464

10. Gill, R. (2012). Media, empowerment, and the 'sexualization of culture' debates. *Sex Roles, 66,* 736–745. doi: 10.1007/s11199-011-0107-1; Wasylkiw, L., & Williamson, M. E. (2012). Actual reports and perceptions of body image concerns of young women and their friends. *Sex Roles, 68,* 239–251. doi: 10.1007-012 -0227-2

11. Clay, D., Vignoles, V., & Dittmar, H. (2005). Body-image and self-esteem among adolescent females: Testing the influence of sociocultural factors. *Journal for Research on Adolescence, 15,* 451–477. doi: 10.1111/j.1532-7795.2005.00107.x; Durkin, S. J., Paxton, S. J., & Sorbello, M. (2007). An integrative model of the impact of exposure to idealized female images on adolescent girls' body satisfaction. *Journal of Applied Social Psychology, 37,* 1092–1117. doi: 10.1111/j.1559-1816 .2007.00201.x; Markey, C. N., & Markey, P. M. (2009). Correlates of young women's desire to obtain cosmetic surgery. *Sex Roles, 61,* 158–166. doi:10.1007/s11199 -009-9625-5

12. Hofschire, L. J., & Greenberg, B. S. (2002). Media's impact on adolescents' body dissatisfaction. In J. D. Brown, J. R. Steele, & K. Walsh-Childers (Eds.) *Sexual Teens, Sexual Media.* Hillsdale, NJ: Erlbaum.

13. Mooney, E., Farley, H., & Strugnell, C. (2009). A qualitative investigation into the opinions of adolescent females regarding their body image concerns and dieting practices in the Republic of Ireland (ROI). *Appetite, 52,* 485–491. doi: 10.1016/j.appet.2008.12.012

14. Hawkins, N., Richards, P. S., Granley, H. M., & Stein, D. M. (2004). The impact of exposure to the thin-ideal media image on women. *Eating Disorders, 12,* 35–50; Monro, F., & Huon, G. (2005). Media portrayed idealized images, body shame, and appearance anxiety. *International Journal of Eating Disorders, 38,* 85–90. doi: 10.1002/eat.20153; Sarwer, D. B., & Crerand, C. E. (2004). Body image and cosmetic medical treatments. *Body Image, 1,* 99–111. doi: http://dx.doi .org/10/1016/S1740-1445(03)00003-2; Stice, E., & Shaw, H. E. (2002). Role of body dissatisfaction in the onset and maintenance of eating pathology: A synthesis of research findings. *Journal of Psychosomatic Research, 53,* 985–993. doi: http://dx .doi.org/10/1016/5O022-3999(02)00488-9; Ward, L. M., & Harrison, K. (2005).

The impact of media use on girls' beliefs about gender roles, their bodies, and sexual relationships: A research synthesis. In E. Cole & J. H. Daniels (Eds.), *Featuring females: Feminist analyses of media* (pp. 3–23). Washington, DC: American Psychological Association.

15. Markey, C. N., & Markey, P. M. (2010). A correlational and experimental examination of reality television viewing and interest in cosmetic surgery. *Body Image, 7,* 165–171. doi: http://dx.doi.org/10.1016/j.body.im.2009.10.006; Markey, C. N., & Markey, P. M. (2012). Emerging adults' responses to a media presentation of idealized female beauty: An examination of cosmetic surgery in reality television. *Psychology of popular media culture, 1,* 209–219. doi: 10.1037/a0027869

16. Schooler, D., Kim, J. L., & Sorsoli, C. L. (2006). Setting rules of sitting down: Parental mediation of television consumption and adolescent well-being. *Sexual Research and Social Policy, 3,* 49–62.

17. Pieters, R., & Wedel, M. (2012). Ad gist: Ad communication in a single eye fixation. *Marketing Science, 31,* 59–73. doi: 10.1287/mksc.1110.0673

18. Norton, K. I., Olds, T. S., Olive, S., & Dank, S. (1996). Ken and Barbie at life size. *Sex Roles, 34,* 287–294. doi: 10.1007.BF01544300

19. Bahadur, N. (2013, July 1). 'Normal' Barbie by Nickolay Lamm shows us what Mattel dolls might look like if based on actual women. *The Huffington Post.* Retrieved from http://www.huffingtonpost.com/2013/07/01/normal-barbie-nickolay-lamm_n_3529460.html

20. Dittmar, H., Halliwell, E., & Ive, S. (2006). Does Barbie make girls want to be thin? The effect of experimental exposure to images of dolls on the body image of 5 to 8 year old girls. *Developmental Psychology, 42,* 286–292. doi: 10.1037/0012-1649.42.2.283

21. Castle, D. J., Honigman, R. J., & Phillips, K. A. (2001). Does cosmetic surgery improve psychosocial well-being? *Medical Journal of Australia, 176,* 601–604.

22. Slater, A., Tiggemann, M., Firth, B., & Hawkins, K. (2012). Reality check: An experimental investigation of the addition of warning labels to fashion magazine images on women's mood and body dissatisfaction. *Journal of Social and Clinical Psychology, 31,* 105–122. doi: 10.1521/jscp.2012.31.2.105

23. Goldwert, L. (2011, June 24). AMA takes stand on Photoshop; Medical association: Altering contributes to unrealistic expectations. *New York Daily News.* Retrieved from http://www.nydailynews.com/life-style/fashion/ama-takes-stand-photoshop-medical-association-altering-contributes-unrealistic-expectations-article-1.126921

24. National Press Photographers Association (2012). *NPAA code of ethics.* Retrieved from https://nppa.org/code-of-ethics

25. Melago, C. (2009, October 24). Ralph Lauren model Filippa Hamilton: I was fired because I was too fat! *New York Daily News.* Retrieved from http://www.nydailynews.com/life-style/fashion/ralph-lauren-model-filippa-hamilton-fired-fat-article-1.381093; Size four model: I was fired for being too fat. (2009, October

14). *Today.* Retrieved from http://www.today.com/id/33307721/ns/today-style/t /size-model-i-was-fired-being-too-fat/#.UWIdqVezfIs

26. Sweeny, M. (2009, December 16). Twiggy's Olay ad banned over airbrushing. *The Guardian.* Retrieved from http://www.guardian.co.uk/media/2009/dec/16 /twiggys-olay-ad-banned-airbrushing

27. Fox, K. R. (1999). The influence of physical activity on mental well-being. *Public Health Nutrition, 3a,* 411–418. doi: http://dx.doi.org/10.1017/S1368980 099000567; Huang, J. S., Norman, G. J., Zabinski, M. F., Calfas, K., & Patrick, K. (2007). Body image and self-esteem among adolescents undergoing an intervention targeting dietary and physical activity behaviors. *Journal of Adolescent Health, 40,* 245–251. doi: http://dx.doi.org/10/1016/j.jadohealth.2006.09.026; Loland, N. W. (1998). Body image and physical activity: A survey among Norwegian men and women. *International Journal of Sport Psychology, 29,* 339–365.

28. Albertini, R. S., & Phillips, K. A. (1999). Thirty-three cases of body dysmorphic disorder in children and adolescents. *Journal of the American Academy of Child and Adolescent Psychiatry, 38,* 453–459. doi: http://dx.doi.org.proxy.libraries.rutgers. edu/10.1097/00004583-199904000-00019; Reas, D. L., & Grilo, C. M. (2004). Cognitive-behavioral assessment of body image disturbances. *Journal of Psychiatric Practice, 10,* 314–322. doi: http://dx.doi.org.proxy.libraries.edu/10.1097/00131746 -200409000-00005

29. Fredrickson, B., Noll, S., Roberts, T., Twenge, J., & Quinn, D. (1998). That swimsuit becomes you: Sex differences in self-objectification, restrained eating, and math performance. *Journal of Personality and Social Psychology, 75,* 269–284; Noll, S. M., & Fredrickson, B. L. (1998). A meditational model linking self-objectification, body shame, and disordered eating. *Psychology of Women Quarterly, 22,* 623–636. doi: 10.1111/j.1471-6402.1998.tb00181.x

30. Wasylkiw, L., & Williamson, M. E. (2012). Actual reports and perceptions of body image concerns of young women and their friends. *Sex Roles, 68,* 239–251. doi: 10.1007-012-0227-2

31. Holsen, I., Jones, D. C., & Birkeland, M. S. (2012). Body image satisfaction among Norwegian adolescents and young adults: A longitudinal study of the influence of interpersonal relationships and BMI. *Body Image, 9,* 201–208. doi: http:// dx.org/10.1016/j.bodyim.2012.01.006; Pearl, R. L., Puhl, R. M., & Brownell, K. D. (2012). Positive media portrayals of obese persons: Impact on attitudes and image preferences. *Health Psychology, 31,* 821–829. doi: 10.1037.a0027189

Chapter 5: Phase Two: Bite by Bite

1. Polivy, J., & Herman, P. C. (2002). If at first you don't succeed: False hopes of self-change. *American Psychologist, 57,* 677–689; Cervone, D., Jirvani, N., & Wood, R. (1991). Goal setting and the differential influence of self-regulatory processes on complex decision making performance. *Journal of Personality and Social Psychology,*

61, 257–266; Foster, G. D., & Kendall, P. C. (1994). The realistic treatment of obesity: Changing the scales of success. *Clinical Psychology Review, 14*, 701–736.

2. Yang, Q. (2010). Gain weight by "going diet?" Artificial sweeteners and the neurobiology of sugar cravings. *Neuroscience, 83*, 101–108; Malik, V. S., Schulze, M. B., & Hu, F. B. (2006). Intake of sugar-sweetened beverages and weight gain: A systematic review. *American Journal of Clinical Nutrition, 84*, 274–288.

3. Fowler, S. P., Williams, K., Resendez, R. G., Hunt, K. J., Hazuda, H. P., & Stern, M. P. (2008). Fueling the obesity epidemic? Artificially sweetened beverage use and long-term weight gain. *Obesity, 16*, 1894–1900; Bray, G. A., Nielsen, S. J., & Popkin, B. M. (2004). Consumption of high-fructose corn syrup in beverages may play a role in the epidemic of obesity. *American Journal of Clinical Nutrition, 79*, 537–543; Gross, L. S., Li, L., Ford, E. S., & Liu, S. (2004). Increased consumption of refined carbohydrates and the epidemic of type 2 diabetes in the United States: an ecologic assessment. *American Journal of Clinical Nutrition, 79*, 774–779.

4. Ogden, C. L., Kit, B. K., Carroll, M. D., & Park, S. (2011). *Consumption of sugar drinks in the United States, 2005–2008*. NCHS Data Brief, 71, 1–8.

5. Chaloupka, F. J., Powell, L. M., & Chriqui, J. F. (2011). Sugar-sweetened beverages and obesity prevention: Policy recommendations. *Journal of Policy Analysis and Management, 30*, 662–664.

6. Gross, L. S., Li, L., Ford, E. S., & Liu, S. (2004) Increased consumption of refined carbohydrates and the epidemic of type 2 diabetes in the United States: An ecologic assessment. *American Journal of Clinical Nutrition, 79*, 774–779.

7. Davis, B., & Carpenter, C. (2009). Proximity of fast food restaurants to schools and adolescent obesity. *American Journal of Public Health, 99*, 505–510.

8. Gardener, H., Rundek, T., Markert, M., Wright, C. B., Elkind, M. S. V., & Sacco, R. L. (2012). Diet soft drink consumption is associated with an increased risk of vascular events in the Northern Manhattan Study. *Journal of General Internal Medicine, 27*, 1120–1126.

9. Heid, M. (2013, March 10). Small snacks curb appetite as well as bigger snacks. *Today Health*. Retrieved from http://www.today.com/health/small-snacks -curb-appetite-well-bigger-snacks-1C8790384?franchiseSlug=todayhealthmain

10. Centers for Disease Control and Prevention (CDC). (2010, September 10). State-specific trends in fruit and vegetable consumption among adults—United States, 2000–2009. *Morbidity and mortality weekly report (MMWR)*. Retrieved from http://www.cdc.gov/mmwr/preview/mmwrhtml/mm5935a1.htm

11. Williams, S. (2014, January 27). Guidelines for men's daily calorie intake. Livestrong. Retrieved from http://www.livestrong.com/article/415222-guide lines-for-mens-daily-calorie-intake/; National Institutes of Health (NIH). (2013, February 13). Balance food and activity. *National Heart, Lung and Blood Institute*. Retrieved from http://www.nhlbi.nih.gov/health/public/heart/obesity/wecan /healthy-weight-basics/balance.htm

12. Smit, H. J., & Rogers, P. J. (2006). Effects of caffeine on mood. In B. D. Smith, U. Gupta, & B. S. Gupta (Eds.), *Caffeine and the activation theory: Effects on health and behavior* (pp. 229–282). Boca Raton, FL: CRC Press; Trayambak, T., Singh, A. L., & Singh, I. L. (2009). Effect of caffeine on vigilance task performance—l: Under low demanding condition. *Indian Journal of Social Science Researchers, 6,* 8–16.

13. Larson, N. I., Nelson, M. C., Neumark-Sztainer, D., Story, M., & Hannan, P. J. (2009). Making time for meals: Meal structure and associations with dietary intake in young adults. *Journal of the American Dietetic Association, 109,* 72–79.

14. Albers, S. (2012). *Eating mindfully: How to end mindless eating and enjoy a balanced relationship with food.* Oakland, CA: New Harbinger.

15. Grotto, D., & Zied, E. (2010). The standard American diet and its relationship to the health status of Americans. *Nutrition in Clinical Practice, 25,* 603–612.

Chapter 6: Get Moving

1. Centers for Disease Control and Prevention (CDC). (2014, June 12). Physical activity facts. Retrieved from http://www.cdc.gov/HealthyYouth/physicalactivity/facts.htm

2. CDC. (2013, April 17). A growing problem. Retrieved from www.cdc.gov/obesity/childhood/problem.html

3. CDC. (2011, March 9). Physical inactivity estimates, by county. Retrieved from http://www.cdc.gov/Features/dsPhysicalInactivity/

4. US Department of Health and Human Services. (2010). *The surgeon general's vision for a healthy and fit nation.* Retrieved from http://www.surgeongeneral.gov/initiatives/healthy-fit-nation/obesityvision2010.pdf

5. Archer, E., Shook, R. P., Thomas, D. M., Church, T. S., Katzmarzyk, P. T., Hebert, J. R., . . . Blair, S. N. (2013). 45-year trends in women's use of time and household management energy expenditure. *PLoS ONE, 8,* e56620. doi:10.1371/journal.pone.0056620

6. Boyland, E. J., Harrold, J. A., Kirkham, T. C., Corker, C., Cuddy, J., Evans, D., . . . Halford, J. C. G. (2011). Food commercials increase preference for energy-dense foods, particularly in children who watch more television. *Pediatrics, 128,* e93-e100. doi: 10.1542/peds.2010-1859

7. CDC. (2014, May 20). Facts about Physical Activity. Retrieved from http://www.cdc.gov/physicalactivity/data/facts.html

8. CDC. (2011, December 1). How much physical activity do adults need? Retrieved from http://www.cdc.gov/physicalactivity/everyone/guidelines/adults.html

9. Knox, O. (2013, February 28). Michelle Obama: Obesity fight is 'generational' campaign. *YahooNews* [blog]. Retrieved from http://news.yahoo.com/blogs/ticket/michelle-obama-obesity-fight-generational-campaign-003906872--election.html

10. CDC (2011, December 1).

11. Ibid.

12. CDC. (1999, November 17). Physical activity and health: A report of the surgeon general. Retrieved from http://www.cdc.gov/nccdphp/sgr/ataglan.htm

13. Hunter, G. R., Bickel, C. S., Fisher, G., Neumeier, W., & McCarthy, J. (2013). Combined aerobic/strength training and energy expenditure in older women. *Medicine & Science in Sports & Exercise, 45,* 1386–1393. doi: 10.1249/MSS.0b013e3182860099

14. CDC. (2009). The power of prevention. Retrieved from www.cdc.gov/chronic disease/pdf/2009-power-of-prevention.pdf

15. Naci, H., & Ioannidis, J. P. A. (2013). Comparative effectiveness of exercise and drug interventions on mortality outcomes: Metaepidemiological study. *British Medical Journal, 347,* f5577. doi: http://dx.doi.org/10.1136/bmj.f5577

16. CDC (2009).

17. Franke, A., Harder, H., Orth, A. K., Zitzmann, S., & Singer, M. V. (2008). Postprandial walking but no consumption of alcoholic digestifs or espresso accelerates gastric emptying in healthy volunteers. *Journal of Gastrointestinal and Liver Diseases, 17,* 27–31; National Institute of Arthritis and Musculoskeletal and Skin Disease. (2009). Exercise for your bone health. Retrieved from http://www.niams.nih.gov/health_Info/Bone/Bone_Health/Exercise/default.asp

18. Baron, K. G., Reid, K. J., & Zee, P. C. (2013). Exercise to improve sleep in insomnia: Exploration of the bidirectional effects. *Journal of Clinical Sleep Medicine, 9,* 819–824. doi: 10.5664/jcsm.2930; Barres, R., Yan, J., Egan, B., Treebak, J. T., Rasmussen, M., Fritz, T., . . . Zierath, J. R. (2012). Acute exercise remodels promoter methylation in human skeletal muscle. *Cell Metabolism, 15,* 405–411. doi: http://dx.doi.org/10.1016/j.cmet.2012.01.001; Reynolds, G. (2013, July 31). How exercise changes fat and muscle cells. *The New York Times* [blog]. Retrieved from http://well.blogs.nytimes.com/2013/07/31/how-exercise-changes-fat-and-muscle-cells/?_php=true&_type=blogs&_php=true&_type=blogs&_r=1&

19. Friedman, H. S., Martin, L. R., Tucker, J. S., Criqui, M. E., Kern, M. L., & Reynolds, C. (2008). Stability of physical activity across the life-span. *Journal of Health Psychology, 13,* 966–978.

20. Gaskins, A. J., Mendiola, J., Afeiche, M., Jorgensen, N., Swan, S. H., & Chavarro, J. E. (2013). Physical activity and television watching in relation to semen quality in young men. *British Journal of Sports Medicine.* doi:10.1136/bjsports-2012-091644

21. Mead, G. E., Morley, W., Campbell, P., Greig, C. A., McMurdo, M., & Lawlor, D. A. (2010). Exercise for depression. New York: John Wiley & Sons. doi: 10.1002/14651858.CD004366.pub5

22. Hoffman, J. (2013, March 8). Exercise may help protect children from stress. *The New York Times* [blog]. Retrieved from http://well.blogs.nytimes.com/2013/03/08/exercise-may-help-protect-children-from-stress/?src=recg

23. Mayo Clinic. (2011, October 1). Depression and anxiety: Exercise eases symptoms. Retrieved from http://www.mayoclinic.com/health/depression-and-exercise/MH00043

24. Blanchfield, A. W., Hardy, J., de Morree, H. M., Staiano, W., & Marcora, S. M. (2013). Talking yourself out of exhaustion: The effects of self-talk on endurance performance. *Medicine & Science in Sports & Exercise, 46*(5): 998–1007. doi: http://dx.doi.org/10.1249/MSS.0000000000000184

25. Reynolds, G. (2013, February 6). Getting into your exercise groove. *The New York Times* [blog]. Retrieved from http://well.blogs.nytimes.com/2013/02/06 /getting-into-your-exercise-groove/?src=me&ref=general

26. Donahue, B. (2013, January 25). How to make an Ironman whimper (and cough). *The New York Times.* Retrieved from http://www.nytimes.com/2013/01/27 /magazine/stair-racing-a-sport-to-make-an-ironman-whimper.html?pagewanted =3&tntemail0=y&_r=0&emc=tnt

27. Vora, S. (2013, April 11). Fitting in at the fitness center. *The New York Times.* Retrieved from http://www.nytimes.com/2013/04/12/nyregion/fitness-centers -friendly-to-out-of-shape-exercisers.html?emc=tnt&tntemail0=y&_r=0

28. Stetler, C. (2013, April 5). Rutgers students use social media to get active. *Rutgers Today.* Retrieved from http://news.rutgers.edu/focus/issue.2013-03-26.832 8999752/article.2013-04-05.4133079037/

29. Reynolds, G. (2013, February 21). The benefits of exercising outdoors. *The New York Times* [blog]. Retrieved from http://well.blogs.nytimes.com/2013/02/21 /the-benefits-of-exercising-outdoors/?ref=health&pagewanted=print

30. Mann, D. (2013, April 30). Sleep and weight gain. *WebMD.* Retrieved from http://www.webmd.com/sleep-disorders/excessive-sleepiness-10/lack-of-sleep -weight-gain

Chapter 7: Phase Three: Eat Smarter

1. US Department of Agriculture (USDA). (2013). Food Groups. *MyPlate.* Retrieved from ChooseMyPlate.gov; BMR calculator: Basal metabolic rate calculator. (n.d.) Myfitnesspal. Retrieved from http://www.myfitnesspal.com/tools/bmr -calculator

2. Young, L. (2013). Food and health with Timi Gustafson: Size matters. Retrieved from http://www.timigustafson.com/2011/size-matters/

3. Michael Pollan and 'In defense of food: The omnivore's solution.' (2008, October 27). *Bates contemplates food.* Retrieved July 25, 2014, http://www.bates.edu /food/foods-importance/omnivores-solution/

4. USDA & US Department of Health and Human Services (1995). Choose a diet low in fat, saturated fat, and cholesterol. *Nutrition and your health: Dietary guides for Americans.* Retrieved from http://www.health.gov/dietaryguidelines/dga95 /lowfat.htm

5. Brown, N. (2013, May 16). How much salt? *The New York Times.* Retrieved from www.newyorktimes.com/2013/05/28/opinion/how-much-salt.html

6. Moss, M. (2013, February 20). The extraordinary science of addictive junk food. *The New York Times Magazine.* Retrieved from http://www.nytimes.com

/2013/02/24/magazine/the-extraordinary-science-of-junk-food.html?ref=magazine&pagewanted=all&_r=0

7. Basu, S., Yoffe, P., Hills, N., & Lustig, R. H. (2013). The relationship of sugar to population level diabetes prevalence: An econometric analysis of repeated cross-sectional data. *PLoS ONE, 8,* 1–8.

8. Lustig, R. H. (2012). *Fat chance: Beating the odds against sugar, processed food, obesity, and disease.* New York: Hudson Street Press.

9. Murphy, M. M., Barraj, L. M., Bi, X., & Stettler, N. (2013). Body weight status and cardiovascular risk factors in adults by frequency of candy consumption. *Nutritional Journal, 12,* 1–11. doi: 10.1186/1475-2891-12-53

10. Sciolino, E. (2013, July 30). A French dining staple is losing its place at the table. *The New York Times.* Retrieved from http://www.nytimes.com/2013/07/31/world/europe/a-french-dining-staple-is-losing-its-place-at-the-table.html?emc=edit_tnt_20130730&tntemail0=y

11. Foster, G. D., Wyatt, H. R., Hill, J. O., Makris, A. P., Rosenbaum, D. L., Brill, C., . . . Klein, S. (2010). Weight and metabolic outcomes after two years on a low-carbohydrate versus low fat diet. *Annuals of Internal Medicine, 153,* 147–157. doi: 10.1059/0003-4819-153-3-201008030-00005

12. Mayo Clinic Staff. (2011). Low carb diet: Can it help you lose weight? Retrieved from www.mayoclinic.com/health/low-carb-diet/NU00279

13. Ibid.

14. Mayo Clinic Staff. (2014, May 2). Carbohydrates: How carbs fit into a healthy diet. Retrieved from www.mayoclinic.com/health/carbohydrates/MY01458

15. USDA. (n.d.). What foods are in the protein foods group? *MyPlate.* Retrieved from http://www.choosemyplate.gov/food-groups/protein-foods.html

16. USDA. (2011). *Eat seafood twice a week.* [PDF]. Retrieved from http://www.choosemyplate.gov/food-groups/downloads/TenTips/DGTipsheet15EatSeafood-BlkAndWht.pdf

17. Mayo Clinic Staff. (2012, November 17). Dietary fiber: Essential for a healthy diet. Retrieved from http://www.mayoclinic.com/health/fiber/NU00033

18. USDA. (n.d.). Grains. *MyPlate.* Retrieved from http://www.choosemyplate.gov/food-groups/grains-why.html

19. Mayo Clinic Staff (2012).

20. USDA. (n.d.). Benefits of breakfast. [PDF]. Retrieved from http://www.fns.usda.gov/sites/default/files/toolkit_benefitsflyer.pdf

21. Gajre, N. S., Fernandez, S., Balakrishna, N., & Vazir, S. (2008). Breakfast eating habit and its influence on attention-concentration, immediate memory, and school achievement. *Indian Pediatrician, 45,* 824–828.

22. Levitsky, D. A., & Pacanowski, C. R. (2013). Effect of skipping breakfast on subsequent energy intake. *Physiological Behavior, 119,* 9–16. doi: 10.1016/j.physbeh.2013.05.006

23. Nocturnal Sleep-Related Eating Disorder. (2011). Anorexia Nervosa and Related Eating Disorders. Retrieved from http://www.anred.com/nsred.html

24. Centers for Disease Control and Prevention. (2013, July 1). How much sleep do I need? Retrieved from http://www.cdc.gov/sleep/about_sleep/how_much_sleep.htm

25. Greer, S. M., Goldstein, A. N., & Walker, M. P. (2013). The impact of sleep deprivation on food desire in the human brain. *Nature Communications, 4*. doi: 10.1038/ncomms3259

26. Young, L. R., & Nestle, M. (2007). Portion sizes and obesity: Responses of fast-food companies. *Journal of Public Health Policy, 28,* 238–248; Nielsen, S. J., & Popkin, B. M. (2003). Patterns and trends in food portion sizes 1977–1998. *Journal of the American Medical Association, 289,* 450–453.

27. Brody, J. (2013, May 20). Many fronts in fighting obesity. *The New York Times* [blog]. Retrieved July 25, 2014, http://well.blogs.nytimes.com/2013/05/20/many-fronts-in-fighting-obesity/?src=recpb

28. Mathias, K. C., Rolis, B. J., Birch, L. L., Kral, T. V., Hanna, E. L., Davey, A., & Fisher, J. O. (2012). Serving larger portions of fruits and vegetables together at dinner promotes intake of both foods among young children. *Journal of the Academy of Nutrition and Dietetics, 112,* 266–270.

29. Wansick, B. (2006). *Mindless eating—why we eat more than we think* (mass market ed.). New York: Bantam Books.

30. Ibid.

31. Disantis, K. I., Birch, L. L., Davey, A., Serrana, E. L., Zhang, J., Bruton, Y., & Fischer, J. O. (2013). Plate size and children's appetite: Effects of larger dishware on self-served portions and intake. *Pediatrics, 131,* 1–8. doi:10.1542/peds.2012-2330

Chapter 8: Restart Smart

1. Polivy, J., & Herman, C. P. (2002). If at first you don't succeed: False hopes of self-change. *American Psychologist, 57,* 677–689.

2. Norcross, J. C., Ratzin, A. C., & Payne, D. (1989). Ringing in the New Year: The change processes and reported outcomes of resolutions. *Addictive Behaviors, 14,* 205–212.

3. Markey, P. M., & Markey, C. N. (2013). Annual variation in internet keyword searches: Linking dieting interest to obesity and negative health outcomes. *Journal of Health Psychology, 18,* 875–886.

4. Jeffrey, R. W., Epstein, L. H., Wilson, T. G., Drewnowski, A., Stunkard, A. J., & Wing, R. A. (2000). Long-term maintenance of weight loss: Current status. *Health Psychology, 19,* 5–16. doi: 10.1037/0278-6133.19.Suppl1.5

5. Anderson, D. (2013, September 10). The do's and don'ts of motivating others. Retrieved from http://coachescoach.biz/the-dos-and-donts-of-motivating-others-by-dean-anderson-behavioral-psychology-expert/

6. Oliver, G., Wardle, J., & Gibson, E. L. (2000). Stress and food choice: A laboratory study. *Psychosomatic Medicine, 62,* 853–865.

7. Rose, N., Koperski, S., & Golomb, B. A. (2010). Mood food: Chocolate and depressive symptoms in a cross-sectional analysis. *Archives of Internal Medicine, 170,* 699–703. doi: 10.1001/archinternmed.2010.78

8. Platte, P., Herbert, C., Pauli, P., & Breslin, P. A. (2013). Oral perceptions of fat and taste stimuli are modulated by affect and mood induction. *PLoS ONE, 8,* e65006. doi:10.1371/journal.pone.0065006

9. Elfhag, K., & Rossner, S. (2005). Who succeeds in maintaining weight loss? A conceptual view of factors associated with weight loss maintenance and weight regain. *Obesity Reviews, 6,* 67–85; Sung, J., Lee, K., Song, Y. M., Lee, M. K., & Lee, D. H. (2010). Heritability of eating behavior assessed using the DEBQ (Dutch Eating Behavior Questionnaire) and weight-related traits: The Healthy Twin Study. *Obesity, 18,* 1000–1005. doi: 10.1038/oby.2009.389

10. Evers, C., Adriaanse, M., de Ridder, D. T., & de Witt Huberts, J. C. (2013). Good mood food: Positive emotion as a neglected trigger for food intake. *Appetite, 68,* 1–7. doi: 10.1016/j.appet.2013.04.007

11. Ibid.

12. van Strien, T., Cebolla, A., Etchemendy, E., Gutierrez-Maldonado, J., Ferrer-Garcia, M., Botella, C., & Baños, R. (2013). Emotional eating and food intake after sadness and joy. *Appetite, 66,* 20–25.

13. Arnow, B., Kenardy, J., & Argas, W. S. (1995). The Emotional Eating Scale: The development of a measure to assess coping with negative affect by eating. *International Journal of Eating Disorders, 18,* 79–90.

14. Ray, C. C. (2013). Analyzing the sweet tooth. *The New York Times.* Retrieved from http://www.nytimes.com/2013/10/15/science/analyzing-the-sweet-tooth .html?emc=edit_tnt_20131014&tntemail0=y

15. Ibid.

16. Mata, J., Todd, P. M., & Lippke, S. (2010). When weight management lasts: Lower perceived rule complexity increases adherence. *Appetite, 54,* 37–43; Shiv, B., & Fedorikhin, A. (1999). Heart and mind in conflict: The interplay of affect and cognition in consumer decision making. *Journal of Consumer Research, 26,* 278–292. doi: 10.1086/209563

17. United States Department of Agriculture (USDA). (2012, October 9). Potatoes. Retrieved from http://www.ers.usda.gov/topics/crops/vegetables-pulses/potatoes .aspx#.Up-IZZTk8Vk

18. Pestano, P., Yeshua, E., & Houlihan, J. (2011, November 20). *Sugar in children's cereals: Popular brands pack more sugar than snack cakes and cookies.* Retrieved from http://www.foodpolitics.com/wp-content/uploads/CEREALSewg_press_cereal _report.pdf

19. By the numbers: What Americans drink in a year. (2011, August 27). *The Huffington Post.* Retrieved from http://www.huffingtonpost.com/2011/06/27/americans -soda-beer_n_885340.html

20. Mata et al. (2010).

21. Foster, G. D., Wadden, T. A., Vogt, R. A., & Brewer, G. (1997). What is a reasonable weight loss? Patients' expectations and evaluations of obesity treatment outcomes. *Journal of Consulting and Clinical Psychology, 65,* 79–85.

22. Whitehead, R. D., Ozakinci, G., & Perrett, D. I. (2013). A randomized controlled trial of an appearance-based dietary intervention. *Health Psychology,* 1–4. doi: 10.1037/a0032322

23. Driver, S., & Hensrud, D. (2013). Financial incentives for weight loss: A one-year randomized controlled clinical trial. Paper presented at the American College of Cardiology 2013 Annual Scientific Sessions, San Francisco.

24. Davidson, A. (2013, March 5). How economics can help you lose weight. *The New York Times.* Retrieved from http://www.nytimes.com/2013/03/10/magazine /how-economics-can-help-you-lose-weight.html?pagewanted=2&src=recg

25. Bennett, G. G., Foley, P., Levine, E., Whiteley, J., Askew, S., Steinberg, D. M., . . . Puleo, E. (2013). Behavioral treatment for weight gain prevention among black women in primary care practice: A randomized clinical trial. *JAMA International Medicine, 173,* 1770–1777. doi: 10.1001/jamainternmed.2013.9263

26. Katz, D. L., & Friedman, R. S. C. (2008). Hunger, appetite, taste, and satiety. In *Nutrition in Clinical Practice* (2nd ed., pp. 377–390). Philadelphia: Lippincott Williams and Wilkins.

27. Izenberg, N. (2013, March 22). Is your kitchen a health hazard? *The New York Times.* Retrieved from http://www.nytimes.com/2013/03/24/opinion/sunday /is-your-kitchen-a-health-hazard.html?emc=tnt&tntemail0=y

28. Andrade, A. M., Greene, G. W., & Melanson, K. J. (2008). Eating slowly led to decreases in energy intake within meals in healthy women. *Journal of the American Dietetic Association, 108,* 1186–1191. doi: 10.1016/j.jada.2008.04.026

29. Otsuka, R., Tamakoshi, K., Yatsuya, H., Murata, C., Sekiya, A., Wada, K., . . . Toyoshima, H. (2006). Eating fast leads to obesity: Findings based on self-administered questionnaires among middle-aged Japanese men and women. *Journal of Epidemiology, 16,* 117–124.

30. Kaipainen, K., Payne, C. R., & Wansink, B. (2012). The mindless eating challenge: Evaluation of a public web-based healthy eating and weight loss program. *Journal of Medical Internet Research, 14,* e168.

31. Bittman, M. (2011, September 25). Is junk food really cheaper? *The New York Times.* Retrieved from http://www.nytimes.com/2011/09/25/opinion/sunday/is-junk -food-really-cheaper.html?pagewanted=all

32. Rolls, B. J., Ello-Martin, M. S., & Tohill, B. C. (2004). What can intervention studies tell us about the relationship between fruit and vegetable consumption and weight management? *Nutrition Review, 62,* 1–17.

33. Ogden, J. (1992). *Fat chance! The myth of dieting explained.* Routledge: New York; McFarlane, T., Polivy, J., & McCabe, R. E. (1999). Help not harm: Psychological foundation for a nondieting approach toward health. *Journal of Social Issues, 55,* 261–276.

34. Ogden, J. (1992); McFarlane et al. (1999).

Chapter 9: Share Your Success and Encourage Others

1. Birch, L. L., & Fisher, J. O. (1998). Development of eating behaviors among children and adolescents. *Pediatrics, 101,* 539–549.

2. Ibid.

3. Ibid.

4. Ogden, J. (2010). *The psychology of eating: From healthy to disordered behavior* (2nd ed.). Chichester, West Sussex, UK: Wiley-Blackwell.

5. Ogden, J., Reynolds, R., & Smith, A. (2006). Expanding the concept of parental control: A role for overt and covert control in children's snacking behaviour? *Appetite, 47,* 100–106. doi: 10.1016/j.appet.2006.03.330

6. Rozin, P., & Tuorila, H. (1993). Simultaneous and temporal contextual influences on food acceptance. *Food Quality and Preference, 4,* 11–20. doi: 10.1016 /0950-3293(93)90309-T

7. Birch & Fisher (1998).

8. Let's move. (n.d.). Retrieved from http://www.letsmove.gov/

9. Taber, D. R., Chriqui, J. F., & Chaloupka, F. J. (2013). State laws governing school meals and disparities in fruit/vegetable intake. *American Journal of Preventive Medicine, 44,* 365–372. doi:10.1016/j.amepre.2012.11.038

10. USDA. (n.d.). MyPlate graphic resources. Retrieved from http://www.choose myplate.gov/print-materials-ordering/graphic-resources.html

11. Harvard School of Public Health. (n.d.). Out with the pyramid, in with the plate. Retrieved from http://www.hsph.harvard.edu/nutritionsource/plate-replaces -pyramid/

12. Lodolce, M. E., Harris, J. L., & Schwartz, M. B. (2013). Sugar as part of a balanced breakfast? What cereal advertisements teach children about healthy eating. *Journal of Health Communication, 18,* 1293–1309. doi: 10.1080/10810 730.2013.778366

13. Bernhardt, A. M., Wilking, C., Adachi-Mejia, A. M., Bergamini, E., Marijnissen, J., & Sargent, J. D. (2013) How television fast food marketing aimed at children compares with adult advertisements. *PLoS ONE, 8,* e72479. doi:10.1371 /journal.pone.0072479

14. Borzekowski, D. L., & Robinson, T. N. (2001). The 30-second effect: An experiment revealing the impact of television commercials on food preferences of preschoolers. *Journal of the American Dietetic Association, 101,* 42–46.

15. Ostroff, J. (2013, March 26). Guilty on junk food. The New York Times. Retrieved from http://www.nytimes.com/2013/03/27/opinion/guilty-on-junk-food .html?src=recpb&_r=0&gwh=38B91AFC36DC1F723E606AB22CFD168D&gwt =pay; Boyland, E. J., Harrold, J. A., Dovey, T. M., Allison, M., Dobson, S., Jacobs, M. C., & Halford, J. C. G. (2013). Food choice and overconsumption: Effect of a premium sports celebrity endorser. *Journal of Pediatrics, 163,* 339–343. doi:10.1016 /j.jpeds.2013.01.059

16. Barnes, B., & Stelter, B. (2013, June 18). Nickelodeon resists critics of food ads. *The New York Times*. Retrieved from http://www.nytimes.com/2013/06/19 /business/media/nickelodeon-resists-critics-of-food-ads.html?nl=todaysheadlines &emc=edit_th_20130619&_r=1&

17. Strom, S. (2013, September 26). With tastes growing healthier, McDonald's aims to adapt its menu. *The New York Times*. Retrieved from http://www.nytimes .com/2013/09/27/business/mcdonalds-moves-toward-a-healthier-menu.html?nl =todaysheadlines&emc=edit_th_20130927&_r=0

18. Strom, S. (2013, September 23). Burger King introducing a lower-fat French fry. *The New York Times*. Retrieved from http://www.nytimes.com/2013/09/24 /business/burger-king-introducing-a-lower-fat-french-fry.html?src=recpb&gwh =AEECC2D34F205D6F7A6222BF445516A9&gwt=pay

19. Nordqvist, C. (2012, June 24). High sugar cereals aggressively marketed at kids, despite pledge. *Medical News Today*. Retrieved from http://www.medicalnews today.com/articles/246996.php

20. Bittman, M. (2013, October 8). Why won't McDonald's really lead? *The New York Times* [blog]. Retrieved from http://opinionator.blogs.nytimes.com/2013 /10/08/why-wont-mcdonalds-really-lead/?nl=todaysheadlines&emc=edit_th _20131009&_r=0

21. Iannotti, R. J., & Wang, J. (2013). Trends in physical activity, sedentary behavior, diet, and BMI among US adolescents, 2001–2009. *Pediatrics, 132,* 606–614. doi: 10.1542/peds.2013-1488

22. Northstone, K., Joinson, C., Emmett, P., Ness, A., & Paus, T. (2012). Are dietary patterns in childhood associated with IQ at 8 years of age? A population-based cohort study. *Journal of Epidemiology and Community Health, 66,* 624–628. DOI: 10.1136/jtech.2010.111955

23. Christakis, N. A., & Fowler, J. H. (2007). The spread of obesity in a large social network over 32 years. *New England Journal of Medicine, 357,* 370–379. doi: 10.1056/NEJMsa066082

24. Markey, C. N., & Markey, P. M. (2014). Gender, sexual orientation, and romantic partner influence on body dissatisfaction: An examination of heterosexual and lesbian women and their partners. *Journal of Social and Personal Relationships.* Vol. 31(2), 162–177. doi:10.1177/0265407513489472

25. Markey, C. N., & Markey, P. M. (2013). Weight disparities between female same-sex romantic partners and weight concerns: Examining partner comparison. *Psychology of Women Quarterly, 37,* 469–477. doi: 10.1177/0361684313484128

26. Markey, C. N., & Markey, P. M. (2011). Romantic partners, weight status, and weight concerns: An examination of the Actor-Partner Interdependence Model. *Journal of Health Psychology, 16,* 217–225. doi: 10.1177/1359105310375636

27. Parker-Pope, T. (2012, April 18). Are most people in denial about their weight? *The New York Times* [blog]. Retrieved from http://well.blogs.nytimes.com /2012/04/18/are-most-people-in-denial-about-their-weight/

28. Loureiro, M. L., & Nayga, R. M. (2006). Obesity, weight loss, and physician's advice. *Social Science and Medicine, 62,* 2458–2468. doi: 10.1016/j.socscimed.2005.11.011

29. Bleich, S. N., Bennett, W. L., Gudzune, K. A., & Cooper, L. A. (2012). National survey of US primary care physicians' perspectives about causes of obesity and solutions to improve care. *BMJ Open, 2,* e001871. doi:10.1136/bmjopen-2012- 001871

30. Loureiro, M. L., & Nayga, R. M. (2006). Obesity, weight loss, and physician's advice. *Social Science and Medicine, 62,* 2458–2468. doi: 10.1016/j.socscimed.2005.11.011

Chapter 10: The Big Picture

1. World Health Organization (WHO). (2010). Urbanization and Health. *Bulletin of the World Health Organization, 88*(4), 245–246. Retrieved from http://www.who.int/bulletin/volumes/88/4/10-010410/en/

2. Centers for Disease Control and Prevention (CDC). (2012, April 27). Overweight and obesity data and statistics. Retrieved from http://www.cdc.gov/obesity/data/index.html

3. US Department of Health and Human Services (USDHHS). (2005, August). *Childhood Obesity.* Retrieved from http://aspe.hhs.gov/health/reports/child_obesity/

4. Pollack, A. (2013, June 18). A.M.A. Recognizes obesity as a disease. *The New York Times.* Retrieved from http://www.nytimes.com/2013/06/19/business/ama-recognizes-obesity-as-a-disease.html?nl=todaysheadlines&emc=edit_th_20130619

5. Centers for Disease Control and Prevention (CDC). (2012, April 27). Overweight and obesity data and statistics. Retrieved from http://www.cdc.gov/obesity/data/index.html

6. CDC. (2012, April 27). Defining obesity. Retrieved from http://www.cdc.gov/obesity/adult/defining.html

7. Olshansky, S. J., Passaro, D. J., Hershow, R. C., Layden, J., Carnes, B. A., Brody, J., . . . Ludwig, D. S. (2012). A potential decline in life expectancy in the United States in the 21st century. *New England Journal of Medicine, 352*(11), 1138–1145. doi: 10.1056/NEJMsr043743; Warner, J. (2010, April 9). Baby boomers may outlive their kids: Higher obesity rates set kids up for poor health. Retrieved from http://www.medicinenet.com/script/main/art.asp?articlekey=115204

8. Ogden, C. L., Carroll, M. D., Kit, B. K., & Flegal, K. M. (2012). Prevalence of obesity and trends in body mass index among US children and adolescents, 1999–2010. *Journal of the American Medical Association, 307,* 483–490. doi: 10.1001/jama.2012.40

9. Ibid.

10. Ogden, C. L., Carroll, M. D., Kit, B. K., & Flegal, K. M. (2014). Prevalence of childhood and adult obesity in the United States, 2011–2012. *Journal of the American Medical Association, 311,* 806–814. doi:10.1001/jama.2014.732

11. Markey, C. N., Markey, P. M., & Schulz, J. (2012). Mothers' own weight concerns predict early child feeding concerns. *Journal of Reproductive and Infant Psychology, 30*(12), 160–167. doi: http://dx.doi.org/10.1080/02646838.2012.693152

12. Ogden et al. (2014).

13. Ervin, R. B., & Ogden, C. L. (2013). Trends in intake of energy and macronutrients in children and adolescents from 1999–2000 through 2009–2010. *NCHS Data Brief, 113*, 1–8.

14. Ibid.

15. WHO. (2009). *Global health risks, mortality and burden of disease attributable to selected major risks.* Retrieved from http://www.who.int/healthinfo/global_burden _disease/GlobalHealthRisks_report_full.pdf

16. Organization for Economic Cooperation Development. (2012). *Obesity Update.* Retrieved from http://www.oecd.org/health/49716427.pdf

17. WHO (2009).

18. Kelland, K. (2012, February 21). Obesity rates in developed countries are rising: Report. *The Huffington Post.* Retrieved from http://www.huffingtonpost.com /2012/02/21/obesity-developedcountries_n_1290937.html

19. Ibid.

20. WHO (2009).

21. National Cancer Institute (2012). Obesity and cancer risk. Retrieved from http://www.cancer.gov/cancertopics/factsheet/Risk/obesity

22. National Institutes of Health (NIH). (2012, July 13). What are the health risks of overweight and obesity? Retrieved from http://www.nhlbi.nih.gov/health /health-topics/topics/obe/risks.html

23. American Heart Association (2014, February 27). Obesity Information. Retrieved from http://www.heart.org/HEARTORG/GettingHealthy/WeightMan agement/Obesity/ObesityInformation_UCM_307908_Article.jsp

24. A codependent relationship: Diabetes and obesity. (n.d.). Retrieved from http://www.diabeticcareservices.com/diabetes-education/diabetes-and-obesity, emphasis mine.

25. Carr, D., Friedman, M. A., & Jaffe, K. (2007). Understanding the relationship between obesity and positive and negative affect: The role of psychosocial mechanisms. *Body Image, 4,* 165–177.

26. Jackson, T. D., Grilo, C. M., & Masheb, R. M. (2000). Teasing history, onset of obesity, current eating disorder psychopathology, body dissatisfaction, and psychological functioning in binge eating disorder. *Obesity Research, 8,* 451–458. doi: 10.1038/oby.2000.56

27. Carr, D., & Friedman, M. A. (2005). Is obesity stigmatizing? Body weight, perceived discrimination, and psychological well-being in the United States. *Journal of Health and Social Behavior, 46,* 244–259.

28. Jackson et al. (2000).

29. Carr & Friedman (2005).

30. Markey, C. N., & Markey, P. M. (2011). Romantic partners, weight status, and weight concerns: An examination of the Actor-Partner Interdependence Model. *Journal of Health Psychology, 16,* 217–225. doi: 10.1177/1359105310375636

31. Alexander, S. C., Coffman, C. J., Tlusky, J. A., Lyna, P., Dolor, R. J., James, I. E., . . . Ostbye, T. (2010). Physician communication techniques and weight loss in adults: Project chat. *American Journal of Preventive Medicine, 39,* 321–328.

32. NIH. (2012, July 13). What causes overweight and obesity? *Health Information for the Public.* Retrieved from http://www.nhlbi.nih.gov/health/health-topics /topics/obe/causes.html

33. Harris, J. L., Bargh, J. A., & Brownell, K. D. (2009). Priming effects of television food advertising on eating behavior. *Health Psychology, 28,* 404–413. doi: 10.1037/a0014399; Lesser, L. I., Zimmerman, F. J., & Cohen, D. A. (2013). Outdoor advertising, obesity, and soda consumption: A cross-sectional study. *BMC Public Health, 13,* 1–7. doi: 10.1186/1471-2458-13-20

34. CDC. (2010). Obesity and genetics. Retrieved from http://www.cdc.gov /features/obesity/

35. Bouchard-Mercier, A., Paradis, A., Rudkowska, I., Lemieux, S., Couture, P., & Vohl, M. (2013). Associations between dietary patterns and gene expression profiles of healthy men and women: A cross-sectional study. *Nutritional Journal, 12,* 1–13. doi: 10.1186/1475-2891-12-24

36. Armon, G., Melamed, S., Shirom, A., Shapira, I., & Berliner, S. (2013). Personality traits and body weight measures: Concurrent and across-time associations. *European Journal of Personality, 27*(4), 398–408. doi: 10.1002/per.1902

37. Kern, M. L., & Friedman, H.S. (2008). Do conscientious individuals live longer? A quanitative review. *Health Psychology, 27,* 505–512. doi: 10.1037/0278 -6133.27.5.505

38. Tucker, J., Friedman, H. S., Tomlinson-Keasey, C., Schwartz, J. E., Wingard, D. L., & Criqui, M. H. (1995). Childhood psychosocial predictors of adulthood smoking, alcohol consumption, and physical activity. *Journal of Applied Social Psychology, 25,* 1884–1899. doi: 10.1111/j.1559-1816.1995.tb01822.x

39. Moss, M. (2013, February 20). The extraordinary science of addictive junk food. *The New York Times.* Retrieved from http://www.nytimes.com/2013/02/24 /magazine/the-extraordinary-science-of-junk-food.html?ref=magazine&pagewanted =all&_r=0

40. Johnson, R. K., Appel, L. J., Brands, M., Howard, B. V., Lefevre, M., Lustig, R. H., . . . Wylie-Rosett, J. (2009). Dietary sugars intake and cardiovascular health. *Circulation, 120,* 1011–1020. doi: 10.1161/CIRCULATIONAHA.109.192627; Everyday-wisdom. (n.d.) Soft drink consumption: The frightening statistics and associated health risks! Retrieved from http://www.everyday-wisdom.com/soft-drink -consumption.html

41. CDC. (2014, May 15). Nutrition services and the school nutrition environment: Results from the School Health Policies and Practices Study 2012. Retrieved from http://www.cdc.gov/HealthyYouth/shpps/index.htm

42. Dermer, M. L., & Jacobson, E. (1986). Some potential negative social consequences of cigarette smoking: Marketing research in reverse. *Journal of Applied Social Psychology, 16,* 702–725. doi: 10.1111/j.1559-1816.1986.tb01754.x

43. Crane, J. K. (2013, March 26). The Talmud and other diet books. *The New York Times.* Retrieved from http://www.nytimes.com/2013/03/27/opinion/the-talmud-and-other-diet-books.html?emc=tnt&tntemail0=y

44. American Heart Association. (2014, July 6). Smoking: Do you really know the risks? Retrieved from http://www.heart.org/HEARTORG/GettingHealthy/Quit Smoking/QuittingSmoking/Smoking-Do-you-really-know-the-risks_UCM_322718 _Article.jsp

45. USDHHS. (2000). *Surgeon general's report on smoking and health.* Washington, DC: Centers for Disease Control and Prevention.

46. Egan, S. (2013, June 25). Why smoking rates are at new lows. *The New York Times* [blog]. Retrieved from http://well.blogs.nytimes.com/2013/06/25/why-smoking-rates-are-at-new-lows/?_php=true&_type=blogs&emc=tnt&tntemail0=y&_r=0

47. Ibid.

48. CDC. (2014, March 28). Adult obesity facts. Retrieved from http://www .cdc.gov/obesity/data/adult.html

49. Rudd Center for Food Policy and Obesity at Yale University. (2008). *Menu labeling in chain restaurants: Opportunities for public policy.* Retrieved from http:// yaleruddcenter.org/resources/upload/docs/what/reports/RuddMenuLabelingReport 2008.pdf

50. Brooks, D. (2013, August 8). The nudge debate. *The New York Times.* Retrieved from http://www.nytimes.com/2013/08/09/opinion/brooks-the-nudge-debate .html?nl=todaysheadlines&emc=edit_th_20130809&_r=0

51. CDC. (n.d.). The facts about obesity. Retrieved from http://www.cdc.gov /pdf/facts_about_obesity_in_the_united_states.pdf

52. Begley, S. (2012, May 1). The costs of obesity. *The Huffington Post.* Retrieved from http://www.huffingtonpost.com/2012/04/30/obesity-costs-dollars-cents_n _1463763.html

53. Campos, P., Saguy, A., Oliver, E., & Gaesser, G. (2006). The epidemiology of overweight and obesity: Public health crisis or moral panic? *International Journal of Epidemiology, 35,* 55–60.

54. Dixon, J. (2013, March 6). Personal Communication.

INDEX

251